Endorsing Institutions

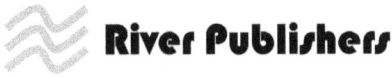

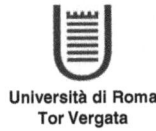

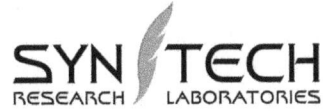

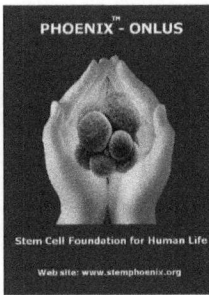

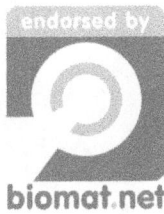

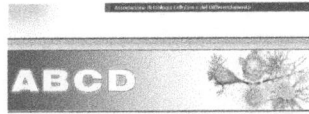

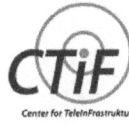

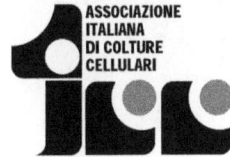

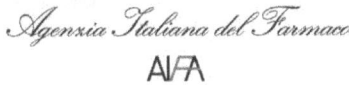

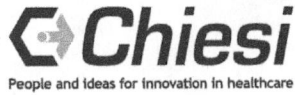

River Publishers

Università di Roma Tor Vergata

SYN TECH RESEARCH LABORATORIES

PHOENIX™ - ONLUS
Stem Cell Foundation for Human Life
Web site: www.stemphoenix.org

endorsed by
biomat.net

ABCD

CTiF
Center for TeleInFrastruktur

ASSOCIAZIONE ITALIANA DI COLTURE CELLULARI

Agenzia Italiana del Farmaco
AIFA

Chiesi
People and ideas for innovation in healthcare

Logistic Partner

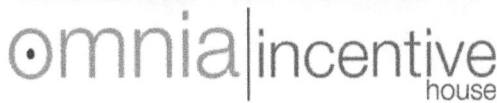

omnia|incentive house

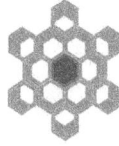

DISPUTATIONES

Adult Progenitor Cells Standardization

Rome, Capitol Hill
1–3 December 2010

www.disputationes.info

Chairman
Paolo Di Nardo

Organised by

River Publishers

Welcome Message from the Chairman

Stem cell research and technology represent a major challenge for treating non-otherwise curable patients. A decade of intensive research has demonstrated that initial hopes based more on enthusiasm than on solid scientific bases can be translated in factual techniques only by adopting more rigorous procedures and strategies. Among other major impediments, the failure so far experienced in applying stem cell technologies to repair parenchymal organs can be ascribed to the lack of sufficient knowledge on basic mechanisms, but also standardized criteria and protocols. Very often, each laboratory follows its own "recipe" using erratic nomenclature and non comparable, if not confusing, experimental protocols. All this makes it difficult to learn from the others and, ultimately, hampers the progression of knowledge on stem cell behaviour.

The ambitious goal of this meeting is to gather the most innovative and scientifically robust knowledge and technologies on stem cells and involve investigators from academy and industry in formulating recommendations to standardize the isolation and manipulation of stem cells using solid and well-documented knowledge rather than fragmentary and often unrepeatable experimental reports.

Paolo Di Nardo (MD)
General Chair — APCS'10
Laboratorio Cardiologia Molecolare & Cellulare
Dip. Medicina Interna
University of Tor Vergata
Via Montpellier, 1 00136
Roma, Italy

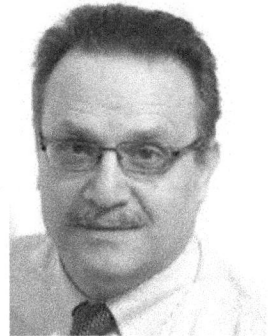

Programme Committee

Luigi Ambrosio

Sebastiano Andò

Luigi Campanella

Sergio Capaccioli

Elisabetta Cerbai

Pier Paolo Di Fiore

Awtar Krishan

Marilena Minieri

Grant Pierce

Maria Prat

Marina Ruggieri

Pawan Singal

Laura Teodori

Organizing Committee

Vincenzo Tavano

Valerio Tavano

Fabio Spadaccini

Mayuri Sinha Prasad

www.disputationes.info

Topics

Round Table 1

Do Adult Progenitor Cells represent a homogeneous population?

Different stem/progenitor cell populations have been identified in various organs. Do these organs really need different systems to repair damaged cells or technical artifacts generate these apparently diverse cell populations?

Round Table 2

Which markers best identify and characterize Adult Progenitor Cells?

Bio-molecular markers are extensively used to identify stem/progenitor cells. However, the markers so far considered are not specific for stem cells and doubts have been cast on some of them about their reliability. Could it be possible to identify arrays of markers capable to identify organ-specific stem/progenitor cells?

Round Table 3

Alternative Strategies to Standardize Progenitor Cells

The different stem/progenitor cells populations could display diversified potency depending on the neighboring microenvironment and, thus, to be prone to preferentially adopt a specific cell phenotype. Could it be possible to setup alternative strategies to identify and characterize them?

Round Table 4

Which strategies to govern Adult Progenitor Cells differentiation?

Different strategies have been described to induce stem/progenitor cells to adopt the same phenotype. This redundancy of *in vitro* differentiating mechanisms could mirror a plethora of mechanisms operating *in vivo*. Nevertheless, in order to promote a harmonic and safe use of stem/progenitor cells for clinical applications, very clearly defined protocols must be setup and validated.

Round Table 5

Is it possible to formulate efficient Adult Progenitor Cell protocols for clinical applications?

Erratic protocols have been so far applied to patients in the need of cell therapy without consistent results. No criteria are available to define the eligibility of a specific patient nor the best conditions to receive cell treatments have been identified. An extensive effort is required to make cell therapy cost-effective.

Scientific Programme Overview

11:00   Registration

1 December 2010

Time: 14:00–16:00
Venue: Round Table, Protomoteca Room, Capitol Hill
Session: Do Adult Progenitor Cells Represent a Homogeneous Population?

16:00–17:00   Opening Ceremony

Venue: Sala della Protomoteca, Capitoline Hill

17:00–17:30   Welcome Party

2 December 2010

Time: 09:30–12:50
Venue: Round Table, Protomoteca Room, Capitol Hill
Session: Which Markers Best Identify and Characterize Adult Progenitor Cells?

12:45–14:10   Lunch

Time: 14:10–17:50
Venue: Round Table, Protomoteca Room, Capitol Hill
Session: Alternative Strategies to Standardize Progenitor Cells

20:00   Visit to the Capitoline Museum Banquet

3 December 2010

Time: 09:15–13:00
Venue: Round Table, Protomoteca Room, Capitol Hill
Session: Which Strategies to Govern Adult Progenitor Cells Differentiation?

12:55–14:20   Lunch

Time: 14:20–16:00
Venue: Round Table, Protomoteca Room, Capitol Hill
Session: Is it Possible to Formulate Efficient Adult Progenitor Cell Protocols for Clinical Applications?

Scientific Programme

11:00 Registration

Time: 14:00–16:00
Venue: Round Table, Protomoteca Room, Capitol Hill
Session: Do Adult Progenitor Cells Represent a Homogeneous Population?
Chair: Awtar Krishan, Maria Prat

14:00–14:20
Adult Stem Cells and Tissue Niche: Two Faces of the Same Medal
Antonio Musarò
Laboratory of Histology and Medical Embryology, University of Rome La Sapienza, Rome, Italy

14:20–14:40
Characteristics of Human Bone Marrow Mesenchymal Stem Cells Culture Amplified Following a Standardized Procedure Set up by the European Project GENOSTEM
Pierre Charbord
INSERM U972, Hôpital de Bicêtre and University Paris 11, Le Kremlin Bicêtre, France

14:40–15:00
Deciphering Cell Fate
Yann Barrandon
Laboratory of Stem Cell Dynamics, School of Life Sciences, Ecole Polytechnique Fédérale Lausanne (EPFL), and Department of Experimental Surgery, Lausanne University Medical School, Lausanne, Switzerland

15:00–15:20
Human Bone-derived Mesenchymal Stem Cells and their Niche
Günter Lepperdinger
Austrian Academy of Sciences, Institute for Biomedical Aging Research, Innsbruck, Austria

15:20–15:40

Understanding Biological Heterogeneity in a Clonal Population of Cells

Michael Halter, Daniel R. Sisan, John T. Elliott, Anne L. Plant

Cell Systems Science Group, Biochemical Science Division, National Institute of Standards and Technology, Gaithersburg, USA

15:40–16:00 Disputatio
16:00–17:00 Opening Ceremony
17:00–17:30 Welcome Party

2 December 2010

Time: 09:30–12:50
Venue: Round Table, Protomoteca Room, Capitol Hill
Session: Which Markers Best Identify and Characterize Adult Progenitor Cells?
Chair: Graham Parker, Laura Teodori

09:30–09:50

Regenerative Potential of the c-kit+AT2+ Precursor Cells

Jun Li

Reference and Translation Center for Cardiac Stem Cell Therapy, University of Rostock, Germany

09:50–10:05

Purinergic Receptor Signaling Varies in Human Mesenchymal and Ectomesenchymal Stem Cell Differentiation

Nina Zippel, Edda Tobiasch

University of Applied Sciences Bonn-Rhein-Sieg, Rhinebach, Germany

10:05–10:20

Should Viral Infectibility be an Additional Required Characteristic of a Deliverable Adult Progenitor Cell?

Barbara Matteoli, Giancarlo Forte, Luca Bontempo, Antonio Scaccino, Antonella Rosati, Enza Fommei, Vittorio Manzari, Marilena Minieri, Paolo Di Nardo, Luca Ceccherini-Nelli

Department of Experimental Pathology, University of Pisa, Pisa, Italy

10:20–10:40 Disputatio
10:40–11:10 Coffee Break

11:10–11:30
Source of Adult Progenitor Cells and their Action
Murli D. Tiwari
Indian Institute of Information Technology, Allahabad, Rajiv Gandhi Institute of Information Technology, Amethi, India

11:30–11:50
Adipose-derived Stem Cells as Source for Tissue Repair and Regeneration
Maria Prat, Andrea Zamperone, Stefano Pietronave
Department of Medical Sciences, University Piemonte Orientale, Novara, Italy

11:50–12:10
Young at Heart: an Update on Progenitor Cells for Cardiac Regeneration
Maria-Jose Goumans
Department of Cardiology, University Medical Center, Utrecht, The Netherlands

12:10–12:25
Mammal Peripheral Blood Stem Cell: Phenotypic Characterization by Cytofluorimetric Analysis
Marco Ranalli, Gabriella Marfè, Gianluca Rotta, Valentina Martini, Marco Polettini, Carla Di Stefano, Paola Sinibaldi-Salimei, Alessandra Gambacurta
Department of Experimental Medicine and Biochemical Sciences, University of Rome Tor Vergata, Rome, Italy

12:25–12:45   Disputatio
12:45–14:10   Lunch

Time: 14:10–17:50
Venue: Round Table, Protomoteca Room, Capitol Hill
Session: Alternative Strategies to Standardize Progenitor Cells
Chair: Murli D. Tiwari, Antonio Musarò

14:10–14:30
The Role of Information and Communication Technology in Cell Standardization
Marina Ruggieri, Alessandro Boni, Tommaso Rossi, Cosimo Stallo
CTIF_Italy, University of Rome Tor Vergata, Rome, Italy

14:30–14:50
How Can Engineers Help?
Arti Ahluwalia
Centro Piaggio, University of Pisa, Pisa, Italy

14:50–15:10

The Ethics of How Stem Cell Research is Represented

Graham Parker

Department of Pediatrics, Wayne State University School of Medicine, Children's Hospital of Michigan, Beaubien, Detroit, USA

15:10–15:25

The Role of Immunosuppression in the Transplantation of Allogenic Neural Precursors Derived from Human Embryonic Stem Cells

Jean Villard

Immunology and Transplant Unit, Geneva University Hospital and Medical School, Geneva, Switzerland

15:25–15:40

Generation of Kit-Egfp ES and EG Cells

Florencia Barrios, Raffaele Geremia, Susanna Dolci

Department of Public Health and Cell Biology, University of Rome Tor Vergata, Rome, Italy

15:40–16:00   Disputatio
16:00–16:30   Coffee Break

16:30–16:45

Cooperation of Biological and Mechanical Signals in Murine Cardiac Progenitor Cell Differentiation

Stefania Pagliari, Ana Cristina Vilela-Silva, Giancarlo Forte, Francesca Pagliari, Corrado Mandoli, Stefano Pietronave, Eugenio Magnani, Giorgia Nardone, Giovanni Vozzi, Arti Ahluwalia, Enrico Traversa, Maria Prat, Marilena Minieri, Paolo Di Nardo

Laboratory of Cellular and Molecular Cardiology, University of Rome Tor Vergata, Rome, Italy

16:45–17:00

Developing an Organotypic *in vitro* 3D Toxicological Test by a Continuous, Stable, non-Tumourogeic Mesenchymal Progenitors Cell Line Derived from the Rat Dental Pulp

Giovanni Berta, Francesca Pagliari, Federica Di Scipio, Stefania Pagliari, Andea Sprio, Paolina Salamone, Eugenio Magnani, Giorgia Nardone, Giancarlo Forte, Paolo Di Nardo

Department of Clinical and Biological Sciences, University of Turin, Turin, Italy

17:00–17:15

Molecular Characterization of Stem Cells in Breast Cancer

Gabriella Di Cola, Leopoldo Sarli, Luigi Roncoroni

European Clinic & Research, Emigroup and University of Parma, Parma, Italy

17:15–17:30

Identification of Circulating Keratinocyte Progenitors and their Differentiation for Potential Application in Skin Tissue Engineering

Lissy K. Krishnan

Sree Chitra Tirunal Institute for Medical Sciences and Technology, Trivandrum, India

17:30–17:50   Disputatio

20:00   Visit to the Capitoline Museum, Banquet

3 December 2010

Time: 09:15–13:00
Venue: Round Table, Protomoteca Room, Capitol Hill
Session: Which Strategies to Govern Adult Progenitor Cells Differentiation?
Chair: Yann Barrandon, Ronglih Liao

09:15–09:35

Adult Human Mesenchymal Stem Cells: Characterization, Differentiation, and Application for Hard and Soft Tissue Regeneration

Lucy di Silvio

Biomaterials Department, King's College Dental Institute, Guy's Hospital, London, United Kingdom

09:35–09:55

Cardiac iPS Cells Repair and Regenerate Infarcted Myocardium

Dinender K. Singla

College of Medicine, Biomolecular Science Center, University of Central Florida, Orlando, USA

09:55–10:10

The Preliminary Portrayal of a Novel Cell-Line Model System for Mouse Cardiac Stem/Progenitor (CSC/CPC) Cells

Ana Freire, Diana S. Nascimento, Giancarlo Forte, Isabel Carvalho, Paolo Di Nardo, Perpetua Pinto do O'

Instituto Nacional de Engenharia Biomédica, Universidade do Porto, Porto, Portugal

10:10–10:25

Strategies to Assist Cell Differentiation, Growth and Direction for Tissue Engineering

Laura Teodori, Dario Coletti, Maria Cristina Albertini, Marco Rocchi, Massimo Fini, Luigi Campanella

ENEA (Agenzia per le Nuove Tecnologie, l'Energia e lo Sviluppo Economicamente Sostenibile), Rome, Italy

10:25–10:40

Osteoblastic Differentiation in a Subpopulation GEO-GR CD45+ Stem Cell-like by Rapamycin Treatment

Gabriella Marfè, Carla Di Stefano, Valentina Martini, Paola Sinibaldi-Salimei, Marco Ranalli, Alessandra Gambacurta

Department of Experimental Medicine and Biochemical Sciences, University of Rome Tor Vergata, Rome, Italy

10:40–11:00   Disputatio
11:00–11:30   Coffee break

11:30–11:45

Characterization of Epithelial Stem Cells, Biomaterials and *in vitro* Microenvironment for Tissue Engineering: Application in Cutaneous Ulcer Therapy

Umberto Altamura, Federico Di Gesualdo, Matteo Lulli, Sergio Capaccioli

Niguarda Hospital, Milan and Department of Pathology, University of Florence, Florence, Italy

11:45–12:00

Considerations about the Controlled Repair of Diseased Renal Parenchyma after Implantation of Stem/Progenitor Cells

Will W. Minuth, Lucia Denk

Molecular and Cellular Anatomy, University of Regensburg, Regensburg, Germany

12:00–12:15

Implantation of Cardiac Stem Cell-loaded poly-Lactic Acid and Fibrinoin Scaffolds into Nude Mice to Evaluate Potential for Cardiac Muscle Tissue Engineering

Valentina Di Felice, Angela De Luca, Claudia Serradifalco, Luigi Rizzuto, Antonella Marino Gammazza, Patrizia Di Marco, Giovanna Cassata, Roberto Puleio, Lucia Verin, Antonella Motta, Annalisa Guercio, Giovanni Zummo

Department BIONEC, University of Palermo, Palermo, Italy

12:15–12:25

A Novel Bioreactor to Mechanically Stress Rat Mesenchymal Stem Cells (MSCs) in Culture

Marco Govoni, Emanuele Giordano, Claudio Muscari, Gianandrea Pasquinelli, Silvio Cavalcanti, Claudio M. Caldarera, Carlo Guarnieri

Dept. Biochemistry "G.Moruzzi", University of Bologna, Bologna, Italy

12:25–12:35
Implantation of Dental Pulp Stem Cells in Isolated Rat Heart in the Absence and in the Presence of Regional Ischemia
Raffaella Rastaldo, Anna Folino, Andrea E. Sprio, Federica Di Scipio, Paolina Salamone, Stefano Geuna, Pasquale Pagliaro, Giovanni N. Berta, Gianni Losano
Department of Clinical and Biological Sciences, University of Turin, Turin, Italy

12:35–12:55   Disputatio
12:55–14:20   Lunch

Time: 14:20–16:00
Venue: Round Table, Protomoteca Room, Capitol Hill
Session: Is it Possible to Formulate Efficient Adult Progenitor Cell Protocols
             for Clinical Applications?
Chair: Maria Jose Goumans, Jun Li

14:20–14:40
Cellular Therapies and Regenerative Medicine Strategies for Diabetes
Camillo Ricordi, Juan Dominguez-Bendala, Armando Mendez, Xiumin Xu, Carlo Tremolada, Luca Inverardi
Diabetes Research Institute and Cell Transplant Center, University of Miami, Miami, USA

14:40–15:00
Adult Stem Cells for Cardiac Repair and Regeneration: Promises and Challenges
Ronglih Liao
Cardiac Muscle Research Laboratory, Brigham and Women's Hospital and Harvard Medical School, Boston, USA

15:00–15:20
Feasibility of Allogeneic Bone Marrow Cells for Cell Therapy to Repair Damaged Myocardium after Myocardial Infarction
Ren-Ke Li
Department of Cardiovascular Surgery, Toronto General Research Institute, Toronto, Canada

15:20–15:40

Generation of Scaffoldless Human Cardiac Patches Using Adult Cardiac Progenitor Cells and Thermo-Responsive Technology

Giancarlo Forte, Stefano Pietronave, Francesca Pagliari, Stefania Pagliari, Eugenio Magnani, Giorgia Nardone, Cristina Giacinti, Antonio Musarò, Enrico Traversa, Teruo Okano, Andrea Zamperone, Marilena Minieri, Maria Prat, Paolo Di Nardo

Laboratory of Cellular and Molecular Cardiology, University of Rome Tor Vergata, Rome, Italy

15:40–16:00 Disputatio
16:00–16:20 Coffee Break

16:20–16:40

Limbal Stem-Cell Therapy and Long-Term Corneal Regeneration

Graziella Pellegrini

University of Modena-Reggio Emilia, Modena, Italy

16:40–17:00

Limbal Cell Therapy for Ocular Surface: A Successful Model of Regenerative Medicine

Geeta K. Vemuganti

Hyderabad Eye Research Centre, LV Prasad Eye Institute, Hyderabad, India

17:00–17:20

Resurgence of Dormant Cancer is an Imperative Consideration in Stem Cell Therapy

Shyam A. Patel, Sarah A. Bliss, Meneke A. Dave, Pranela Rameshwar

Dept. of Medicine-Hematology/Oncology, New Jersey Medical School, Newark, USA

17:20–17:35

Immortalized Bone Marrow-Derived Mesenchymal Stromal Cells Promote Axonal Survival in a Mouse Model of Krabbe's Disease

Caterina Miranda, Carla Teixeira, Marcia Liz, Vera Sousa, Filipa Franquinho, Giancarlo Forte, Paolo Di Nardo, Perpetua Pinto do O', Monica Mendes Sousa

Nerve Regeneration Group, Institute for Molecular and Cell Biology, Porto, Portugal

17:35–17:45

Preliminary Studies on the Production of Canine Mesenchymal Stem Cells from Adipose Tissue and Possible Applications in Dogs with Orthopaedic Lesions

Patrizia Di Marco, Valentina Di Felice, Giuseppa Purpari, Vincenza Cannella, Samanta Partanna, Santina Di Bella, Annalisa Guercio

Istituto Zooprofilattico Sperimentale della Sicilia "A. Mirri", Palermo, Italy

17:45–17:55
Digging and Drawing Cardiac Progenitor Cell (CPCs) Response(s) to Heart Injury
Diana S. Nascimento, M. Valente, Ana Freire, Sofia Correia, Isabel Carvalho, Perpetua Pinto do O'
Instituto Nacional de Engenharia Biomédica, Universidade do Porto, Porto, Portugal

17:55–18:15   Disputatio

Closing Remarks

Abstracts

Time: 14:00–16:00
Venue: Round Table, Protomoteca Room, Capitol Hill
Session: Do Adult Progenitor Cells Represent a Homogeneous Population?
Chair: Awtar Krishan, Maria Prat

14.00–14.20

ADULT STEM CELLS AND TISSUE NICHE: TWO FACES OF THE SAME MEDAL

Antonio Musarò
DAHFMO-Unit of Histology and Medical Embryology Sapienza University of Rome, Italy

One of the most exciting aspirations of current medical science is the regeneration of damaged body parts. The capacity of adult tissues to regenerate in response to injury stimuli represents an important homeostatic process. Regeneration of adult skeletal muscle is a highly coordinated program that partially recapitulates the embryonic developmental program. However, muscle regeneration is affected in several pathological conditions. Although stem cell therapy has not yet solved the major problem related to cell transplantation, namely the capacity to survive and to improve muscle regeneration, recent studies are beginning to elucidate the signals and mechanisms whereby regenerating muscle recruits circulating cells to sites of injury or degeneration. These cells need not be stem cells as long as they maintain sufficient plasticity to participate in muscle repair, either by rebuilding the damaged tissue or by instructing resident precursors.

Thus, one of the crucial parameters of tissue regeneration is the microenvironment in which the stem cell populations should operate. Stem cell microenvironment, or niche, provides essential cues that regulates stem cell proliferation and that directs cell fate decisions and survival.

It is therefore plausible that loss of control over these cell fate decisions might lead to a pathological transdifferentiation or cellular transformation. Current advances in stem cell biology justify a cautious optimism, yet the presence of stem cells seems to be not sufficient to guarantee an efficient tissue regeneration and repair. Specific factors are required to trigger stem cells toward a specific lineage, to improve their survival, and to render them effective in contributing to tissue repair. Studies on stem cell niche leaded to the identification of critical players and physiological conditions that improve tissue regeneration and repair.

Among these, insulin-like growth factor (IGF-1) has been involved in the modulation of inflammatory response and in the regulation of muscle regeneration and homeostasis.

These evidences suggest that while stem cells represent an important determinant for tissue regeneration, a "qualified" environment is necessary to guarantee and achieve functional results.

14.20–14.40

CHARACTERISTICS OF HUMAN BONE MARROW MESENCHYMAL STEM CELLS CULTURE-AMPLIFIED FOLLOWING A STANDARDIZED PROCEDURE SET UP BY THE EUROPEAN PROJECT GENOSTEM

Pierre Charbord

INSERM U972, Hôpital de Bicêtre, and University Paris 11, Le Kremlin Bicêtre, France

Genostem (acronym for "Adult mesenchymal stem cells engineering for connective tissue disorders. From the bench to the bed side") has been an European consortium of 30 teams working together on human bone marrow Mesenchymal Stem Cell (MSC) biological properties and repair capacity. The consortium has set up a standardized protocol for the culture of human bone marrow MSCs. Standards for the culture system included the use of alpha-MEM (without nucleotides) and of fetal calf serum selected for cell growth (from Hyclone^R), and a cell seeding concentration of 5×10^4 cells/cm^2 at culture initiation and of 10^3/cm^2 at each passage. Fibroblast growth factor-2 (FGF-2) was added at low concentration (1 ng/mL twice a week at medium renewal) in culture of elderly patients. We have shown that culture-amplified, clonogenic and highly-proliferative MSCs were bona fide stem cells, that shared with other stem cell types the major attributes of self-renewal, multipotentiality and of multi-potential priming to the lineages to which they can differentiate (osteoblasts, chondrocytes, adipocytes and vascular smooth muscle cells/pericytes). Extensive study of membrane antigens has shown that MSCs constituted an heterogeneous population of immature cells, clearly distinct from other bone cell types of either hematopoietic or mesenchymal origin. Some of the antigens detected on culture-amplified cells were also useful for the isolation of native bone marrow cells. Finally and most importantly, we have shown that locally implanted MSCs effectively repair bone, cartilage and tendon. This study indicates that it is possible to formulate efficient adult stem/progenitor cell protocols for clinical applications.

14:40–15:00

DECIPHERING CELL FATE

Yann Barrandon

Laboratory of Stem Cell Dynamics, School of Life Sciences, Ecole Polytechnique Fédérale Lausanne (EPFL), and Department of Experimental Surgery, Lausanne University Medical School, Lausanne, Switzerland.

Regenerative medicine holds great expectations and reprogramming cell fate is a promising route to reconstructing tissue or organ function. Recent reports have demonstrated that reprogramming can be readily achieved by manipulating the genome, usually with a combination of specific transcriptions factors. This can result in lineage conversion up to ground pluripotent embryonic state. However, regulatory constraints will certainly impact the genetic approach, and consequently translation to clinic may be difficult. An alternate route is to manipulate the microenvironment, and we have recently demonstrated that thymic epithelial cells can acquire the functionality of multipotent stem cells of the skin when exposed to appropriate microenvironmental cues (Bonfanti et al., Nature 2010). Therefore, many routes must be simultaneously explored to successfully bring regenerative medicine from bench to bedside.

15:00–15:20

HUMAN BONE-DERIVED MESENCHYMAL STEM CELLS AND THEIR NICHE
Günter Lepperdinger
Austrian Academy of Sciences, Institute for Biomedical Aging Research, Innsbruck, Austria

Stem cells are vitally involved in tissue regeneration and homeostasis in late life. Mesenchymal stem cells (MSC) (also known as multipotent stromal progenitor cells) are but one particular type of the so-called tissue-specific (or adult) stem cells. Yet this stem cell type appears to be particularly interesting as MSC can differentiate into many different types of mesoderm derivative. Upon stimulation (e.g. injury), stem cells nesting in their niche commence proliferation thereby giving rise to one stem cell (self-renewal) and one progenitor cell, which proliferates further on. Progeny of the latter differentiates to regain functional mesenchymal tissue. In order to insure tissue maintenance, each of these processes has to be tightly regulated.

Tissue aging is paralleled by the loss of tissue regeneration capacity and thus a decline in function. Yet loss of tight control is often observed at advancing age, and this arising deficit may eventually lead to accumulation of fat deposits in bone, impaired fracture healing, deregulated hematopoiesis, and autoimmunity.

Provided that there are two fundamental questions in the field, which need to be addressed in order to reach a decision, which is the best stem cell source for subsequent biomedical applications: (i) how to select high quality MSC with respect to proliferation capacity and differentiation potential as well as their ability to suppress the activation of immune cells; (ii) what are valid markers and standardized conditions regarding the in vitro propagation of MSC for the purpose of tissue engineering and immune modulation therapy.

These two problems share one commonality which actually relates to the in vivo niche: specification and maintenance of stemness cells take place in distinct sites within the body. Meanwhile, relatively little is known about the MSC niche and even less understood are those instructive measures of the niche, which assure life-long stemness of MSC. In this contribution we will outline biological cues that are crucial for MSC stemness such as oxygen tension, domineering bioactive factors and regulative neuroendocrine stimuli. At last, age-associated changes are put forward which eventually lead to sustaining alterations within the putative MSC niche.

15:20–15:40

UNDERSTANDING BIOLOGICAL HETEROGENEITY IN A CLONAL POPULATION OF CELLS

Michael Halter, Daniel R Sisan, John T Elliott and Anne L Plant
Cell Systems Science Group, Biochemical Science Division, National Institute of Standards and Technology, Gaithersburg, USA

A population of cells in culture displays a range of phenotypic responses, even when those cells are genetically identical. The extent of variation in phenotype depends on the phenotypic response being observed. Variations in cell volumes, which we have shown to be the result of differences in cell growth rates and division times across the population, take the shape of a nearly Gaussian distribution, while distributions in the activity of the promoter for the extracellular matrix protein tenascin-C are highly non-Gaussian and are characterized by a significantly larger coefficient of variation, indicating a larger amount of heterogeneity. We have taken several experimental and theoretical approaches to understand this heterogeneity as a result of stochastic fluctuations in intracellular biochemical reactions. Stationary distributions of population phenotypes have been measured by flow cytometry and by imaging of fixed cells. Live cell microscopy of GFP expression over long periods of time has allowed us to track time-dependent promoter activity in individual cells and their offspring. Using Fluorescence Activated Cell Sorting we can separate a population of cells with low tenascin promoter activity from a population of high promoter activity, and monitor the two populations as they relax back to the original distribution of GFP intensities. We observe that high and low GFP expressing populations return to the steady state distribution with different rates. Using kinetic parameters derived from both the live cell imaging data and the relaxation experiments, we infer the contribution that stochastic components are making on the tenascin-C gene expression distributions, and can hypothesize about the mechanisms of control of the tenascin-C gene. Understanding the source of biological variability, and careful measurement of biological variability, is critical for distinguishing when differences between cells reflect stochastic fluctuations within a population, and when two populations are truly different from one another.

15:40–16:00   **Disputatio**
16:00–17:00   **Opening Ceremony**
17:00–17:30   **Welcome Party**

December 2, 2010

Time: 09:15–12:50
Venue: Round Table, Protomoteca Room, Capitol Hill
Session: Which Markers Best Identify and Characterize Adult Progenitor Cells?
Chair: Graham Parker, Laura Teodori

09:15–09:35

STEM CELL MARKERS IN CELLS FROM BODY CAVITY FLUIDS

Awtar Krishan
Pathology Department, University of Miami School of Medicine, Miami, USA

Several recent studies have focused on the presence and importance of human tumor stem cells. Expression of cell surface markers (e.g., CD44, CD133), certain detoxifying enzymes (e.g., aldehyde dehydrogenase 1, ALDH1) and drug efflux characteristics (Side Population or SP phenotype) have been used to identify and sort tumor stem cells for growth in vitro and for tumorigenicity in immunodeficient mice. Although expression of specific tumor stem cell markers has been described in a variety of solid tumors, there are few published reports on the expression of these markers in cells from peritoneal or pleural effusions of patients suspected to have a malignancy. In the present report, we have used multiparametric laser flow cytometry to detect cells with tumor stem cell marker expression in peritoneal and pleural effusions of 29 female patients. Our preliminary findings indicate that a high percentage of Ber-EP4 cells in effusions of female patients with malignant and benign disease express markers characteristic of tumor stem cells. The mean and standard deviation of the percent Ber-EP4 cells in the malignant and benign samples was 36.53 ± 27.11 and 26.73 ± 20.69, respectively. In contrast, no major difference in the mean percent of Ber-EP4 cells with CD44/CD24 or CD44/CD24 expression was seen in cells from the malignant and the benign samples. Expression of the so called tumor stem cell markers in cells from some effusions in which diagnostic cytology had not found any malignant cells suggests that either these markers are also expressed by cells other than tumor stem cells or routine cytomorphologic examination of body cavity fluids by diagnostic cytology is not sensitive enough to detect tumor stem cells.

09:35–09:55

REGENERATIVE POTENTIAL OF THE c-kit+AT2+ PRECURSOR CELLS

Jun Li
Reference and Translation Center for Cardiac Stem Cell Therapy, University of Rostock, Germany

Angiotensin II can interfere with cardiac remodelling process via its receptor subtypes, AT1 and AT2 receptor. The expression pattern of AT2 receptor with predominance in less differentiated mesenchymal cells during fetal life and upregulation under pathological conditions during tissue injury/repair process indicates that AT2 receptor may exert an important action in adaptive tissue regeneration, which may be different from the known AT1 receptor-mediated effects of angiotensin II. We have recently defined the c-kit+AT2+ precursor cells in the heart and bone marrow, which increase in response to acute ischemic heart injury in rats. In addition, we have provided evidence that AT2 receptor activation enhances cardiac homing of the c-kit+AT2+ precursor cells, contributing to improved cardiomyocyte performance. Thus far our current data reveal further regenerative potentials of the c-kit+AT2+ precursor cells.

09:55–10:10

PURINERGIC RECEPTOR SIGNALING VARIES IN HUMAN MESENCHYMAL AND ECTOMESENCHYMAL STEM CELL DIFFERENTIATION

Nina Zippel, Edda Tobiasch
University of Applied Sciences Bonn-Rhein-Sieg, Rhinebach, Germany

Purinergic receptors are well known to participate in important cellular processes, such as proliferation and migration, but the role of these receptors during mesenchymal differentiation has been deciphered only fragmentarily so far. Human adult mesenchymal stem cells (MSCs) are of major interest for Regenerative Medicine, in particular due to their ability to differentiate into cells forming muscle, cartilage or bone. In contrast to this, the ectomesenchymal stem cells derived from dental follicle are further committed towards hard tissues. To evaluate the potential influence of P2 receptors in stem cell differentiation, these two stem cell types with their differences in lineage potential have been compared for the receptor expression. The role of metabotropic P2Y and ionotropic P2X receptor subtypes has been examined in mesenchymal and ectomesenchymal stem cells during differentiation and calcium imaging following agonist stimulation was used to demonstrate the functional activity of P2 receptors. Both cell types expressed several functionally active P2X and P2Y receptor subtypes, but with differences in the expression level. Interestingly, some particular P2 receptor subtypes were found to be differently regulated during adipogenic and osteogenic differentiation. Moreover, the administration of agonists and antagonists of P2 receptors had a direct influence on those differentiations. Taken together, purinergic receptors play an important role during the differentiation towards the adipogenic and osteogenic lineage. Thus, in the future, artificial P2 receptor ligands might be used to control mesenchymal stem cell fate.

10:10–10:25

Luca Ceccherini-Nelli
Department of Experimental Pathology, University of Pisa, Pisa, Italy

10:25–10:45   Disputatio
10:45–11:15   Coffee Break

11:15–11:35

SOURCE OF ADULT PROGENITOR CELLS AND THEIR ACTION

Murli D Tiwari
Indian Institute of Information Technology, Allahabad
Rajiv Gandhi Institute of Information Technology, Amethi, India

Pluripotent stem cells can be found in a number of tissues, including umbilical cord blood. Using genetic reprogramming, pluripotent stem cells equivalent to embryonic stem cells have been derived from human adult skin tissue. Other adult stem cells are multipotent, meaning they are restricted in the types of cell they can become, and are generally referred by their tissue of origin. Defining the events in progenitor cells homing and differentiation may enable novel therapeutic strategies to improve or block vasculature regeneration. Homing is multi-step cascade including the initial adhesion to activated endothelial or exposed matrix, transmigration through the endothelium, and finally, migration and invasion into the target tissue. CD34+, bone marrow–derived progenitor cells, contribute to tissue repair by differentiating into endothelial cells, vascular smooth muscle cells, hematopoietic cells, and possibly other cell types. However, the mechanisms by which circulating progenitor cells home to remodeling tissues remain unclear. It has been shown by various scientists that integrin $\alpha 4\beta 1$ (VLA-4) promotes the homing of circulating progenitor cells to the $\alpha 4\beta 1$ ligands VCAM and cellular fibronectin, which are expressed on actively remodeling neovasculature. Progenitor cells, which express integrin $\alpha 4\beta 1$, homed to sites of active tumor neovascularization but not to normal nonimmune tissues. Antagonists of integrin $\alpha 4\beta 1$, but not other integrins, blocked the adhesion of these cells to endothelia in vitro and in vivo as well as their homing to neovasculature and outgrowth into differentiated cell types. These studies describe an adhesion event that facilitates the homing of progenitor cells to the neovasculature.

11:35–11:55

ADIPOSE-DERIVED STEM CELLS AS SOURCE FOR TISSUE REPAIR AND REGENERATION

Maria Prat, Andrea Zamperone, Stefano Pietronave
Department of Medical Sciences, University Piemonte Orientale, Novara, Italy

Cardiac stem cell niche has been defined as a critical microenvironment in which mechano-physical, biochemical and biological factors concur to preserve resident stem cells in their undifferentiated state. The exhaustive identification of such signals remains among the hot topics in stem cell biology. The generation of an artificial niche in vitro relies, in fact, on the definition of the most appropriate biocompatible, biodegradable scaffold that favours, in combination with specific biochemical factors, stem cell growth and differentiation. The mechano-physical features of biocompatible scaffolds elicit *per se* effects on stem cell determination. We show here that 3D scaffolds can enhance the cardiomyogenic potential of cardiac resident Sca-1$^+$ progenitor cells. In particular, we demonstrate that Sca-1$^+$ stem cell differentiation is achieved within a few days when a complex cardiogenic microenvironment is provided by coupling the biological factors arising from neonatal cardiomyocytes and 3D scaffolds that has cardiac-like stiffness. Challenging the cardiac progenitors only with the appropriate tissue-specific scaffolds merely induced the expression of cardiomyocyte-specific proteins without the assembly of sarcomeres, while the complete differentiation of stem cells in co-culture with neonatal cardiomyocytes in conventional 2D conditions required a longer time. In conclusion, our study provides a further and compelling evidence that cardiac progenitor fate can be tuned by a strict combination of biological and physical factors and encourage in vivo studies to investigate the possibility of using 3D poly lactic acid (PLA) scaffolds to fabricate stem cell-derived cardiac patches.

11:55–12:15

YOUNG AT HEART: AN UPDATE ON PROGENITOR CELLS FOR CARDIAC REGENERATION

Maria-Jose Goumans
Department of Cardiology, University Medical Center, Utrecht, The Netherlands

Cardiovascular disease is one of the most important causes of mortality. Important advances have been made in the prevention and treatment of acute complications after myocardial infarction (MI), over the past decade. This has lead to a decrease in the number of deaths in patients with acute MI. However, current treatments can not prevent the loss of cardiac contractility caused by cardiomyocyte death, and therefore patients that do survive MI are prone to develop progressive impaired cardiac function, which may lead to heart failure. Cell-based therapy has been proposed as a potential new therapy to prevent progression to end-stage heart failure by (re)generating contractile tissue in the damaged heart. During the last years, many different cell sources have been studied extensively for their cardiomyogenic differentiation capacity in vivo and in vitro. These cells include several populations of cardiac-derived progenitor cells as well as mesenchymal stem cells derived from different sources. It has become clear that not only the origin, but also the "age" of a cell is an important determinant of its plasticity. Therefore, special attention is paid to the difference in developmental state of the cell sources and the consequences for their differentiation capacity and therapeutic applicability.

12:15–12:30

MAMMAL PERIPHERAL BLOOD STEM CELL: PHENOTYPIC CHARACTERIZATION BY CYTOFLUORIMETRIC ANALYSIS

Marco Ranalli, Gabriella Marfè, Gianluca Rotta, Valentina Martini, Marco Polettini, Carla Di Stefano, Paola Sinibaldi-Salimei, Alessandra Gambacurta
Department of Experimental Medicine and Biochemical Sciences, University of Rome Tor Vergata, Rome, Italy

Studies have shown that the phosphoinositide 3-kinase (PI3K) pathway plays important roles in proliferation, survival and maintenance of pluripotency in human embryonic stem cell (hESCs) Inhibition of mammalian target of rapamycin (mTOR) signalling by rapamycin suppresses the proliferation of mESCs. Rapamycin's contribution to osteogenic differentiation has been demonstrated in various cell types, but the effect of rapamycin on the osteogenic differentiation of hESCs has not been addressed to date.

In this study, we showed that the treatment with rapamycin (a mTOR inhibitor) induced osteoblastic differentiation in subpopulation stem cell like CD45+, (obtained from getifinib resistant GEO colon cell line GEO-GR). In addition, we report that the mTOR inhibitor rapamycin is capable of differentiating this cells toward an osteoblastic phenotype by blocking p70S6K.

Methods

GEO colon carcinoma cell lines were obtained from the American Type Culture Collection. GEO-GR (Gefitinib resistant), cells were established as previously described (Bianco *et al.*, 2008). Stem cell like CD45+ subpopulation were selected from GEO-GR by sorting on a BD FACSAria II flow cytometer.

Results

The subpopulation of stem cells like CD45+, obtained from GEO-GR was cultured in osteogenic differentiation media containing rapamycin at the concentration 10 μM. After seven day of culture, 90% of cells presented typical osteoblastic cell morphology, as shown by the expression of osteoblastic marker protein (osteocalcin). Lysates from undifferentiated stem cells like CD45+ (GEO-GR) and inhibitor-treated stem cells like CD45+ (GEO-GR), were analyzed by western blotting using antibodies against p70S6K, phospho-p70S6K (p-p70S6K), and β-actin (as a loading control). Results showed that undifferentiated stem cells like CD45+ expressed active components of the mTOR pathway, such as p-p70S6.

Conclusion

We conclude that inhibition of PI3K-AKT-mTOR signaling by rapamycin contributes to stem cells like CD45+ (GEO-GR) commitment into osteoblastic lineages in vitro and, therefore, present rapamycin as a new osteogenic factor that stimulates the osteoblastic differentiation of this kind of stem cells.

12:30–12:50   **Disputatio**
12:50–14:10   **Lunch**

Time: **14:10–17:50**
Venue: **Round Table, Protomoteca Room, Capitol Hill**
Session: **Alternative Strategies to Standardize Progenitor Cells**
Chair: **Murli D Tiwari, Antonio Musarò**

14:10–14:30

THE ROLE OF INFORMATION AND COMMUNICATION TECHNOLOGY IN CELL STANDARDIZATION
Marina Ruggieri, Alessandro Boni, Tommaso Rossi, Cosimo Stallo
CTIF_Italy, University of Rome Tor Vergata, Rome, Italy

In the last decades, the progress in the field of Information and Communication Technology (ICT) has been extraordinary. Today, ICT can be considered mature and, therefore, ready to crossfertilize other areas where its technological, modeling and architectural results can be effectively utilized.

Many research fields directly related with the improvement of the Quality of Life (QoL) of human beings can take great advantage from the maturity of ICT.

The Center for TeleInFrastructures (CTIF), a worldwide research network focused on ICT systems and applications, and, in particular, its Italian node (CTIF_Italy) are addressing deep efforts in the use of ICT for improving the QoL, through an interdisciplinary research that, so far, deals with the following fields: Energy, Geology and Biotechnology.

In the latter field, in particular, the focus is on the application of ICT to Stem Cell systems. There are four topics that are being investigated by CTIF_Italy:

i) Modeling Tools for Stem Cells Interaction in Bio-active Scaffolds:

Game Theory (GT) has been widely used in wireless technologies to model medium access, power control or resource exchange. In order to have a wider vision of the problem and describe the evolution of such networks, Evolutionary Game Theory (EGT) is currently considered as an important tool. We applied the theory to study how a stem cells population becomes a myocardial tissue.

ii) Application of Information Theory to Communications between Stem Cells

The aim is to apply the concepts of information theory to the mathematical modeling of the natural reciprocal interaction between cells, in particular between cells and extracellular matrix, with the aim to gain the required knowledge to mediate and regulate this process.

iii) Networking between Biotech Laboratories

INBA (Infrastructural Network for Biotech Advancement) aims at the development of a networking environment for the cooperation of biotech scientists and experts who aim at interacting remotely through tele-measurements and tele-experimental sessions, software driven procedures, advanced web applications in a secure environment.

iv) Secure and Intelligent Database Architectures

Artificial intelligence techniques can be useful tools to realize an intelligent database engine hybrid architecture for data concerning the interaction between cell/scaffold and cell/cell. The intelligent database engine architecture should satisfy specific system security requirements.

In the presentation, the ICT vs QoL framework will be described, along with its application in an interdisciplinary approach. In particular, some of the results achieved so far in the application of ICT to stem cells will be reported.

14:30–14:50

HOW CAN ENGINEERS HELP?
Arti Ahluwalia
Centro Piaggio, University of Pisa, Pisa, Italy

Centro Interdipartimentale di Ricerca "E.Piaggio", University of Pisa.

Stem cells are inherently unstable and their fate in vivo is modulated by the so-called "niche", an anatomic and functional unit in which the unstable stem cells are confined in a semi-quiescent state. Once stem cells are placed in an in-vitro context they are bombarded by a multitude of confounding signals from culture media, serum, and enzymes to pipette tips, petri dishes and CO_2 incubators, many of which are difficult to define, quantify or measure. Not surprisingly a plethora of factors which influence lineage specification have been identified, and on perusing the latest literature reports one gets the impression that if you say "boo" to a stem cell, it differentiates.

In this sense, this workshop comes at a critical moment; as far as in-vitro strategies for controlling the differentiation cascade are concerned we are still groping in the dark. How can engineers help to control the stem cell arena once cells are removed from the in-vivo niche? We need to break down the hopelessly complex in-vivo environment into specific and controllable features and reconstruct these systematically in-vitro. Engineers have a myriad of tools and devices which are underused and unexplored by biologists and clinicians. Amongst these are computational and analytical models, biomaterial and biomaterial processing methods and well-characterised cell culture environments or bioreactors. My argument is that biologists should adopt these tools on a routine basis to enable firstly a global level of standardization of cell culture protocols and cell handling procedures. Secondly, together scientists should assemble well-structured experimental paradigms which allow piecewise and controlled reconstruction of a cell microenvironment. Thirdly, all knowledge acquired should be collated to create a World Databank with the aim of constructing n-dimensional representations of cell response to micro-environmental factors.

14:50–15:10

THE ETHICS OF HOW STEM CELL RESEARCH IS REPRESENTED
Graham Parker
Department of Pediatrics, Wayne State University School of Medicine, Children's Hospital of Michigan, Beaubien, Detroit, USA

Stem cell research and its communication have become, for better and worse, a matter of great public interest. The peer review process is still alive and well, but has taken a severe beating of late. This presentation will touch on some delicate issues relevant to the process, such as motivation behind paper submission, reviewer recommendation and selection. Stem cell researchers are a truly an international community, although communication is primarily in English. However, in spite of international recognition of the importance of ethics in the research and publication process, cultural and regulatory differences create a gulf of perspective that warrants consideration.

15:10–15:25

THE ROLE OF IMMUNOSUPPRESSION IN THE TRANSPLANTATION OF ALLOGENIC NEURAL PRECURSORS DERIVED FROM HUMAN EMBRYONIC STEM CELLS
Jean Villard
Immunology and Transplant Unit, Geneva University Hospital and Medical School, Switzerland

Neural Progenitor Cells (NPC) from a fetal origin or from human embryonic stem cells (hESC) have the potential to differentiate into mature neurons after transplantation into the brain, opening the possibility of regenerative cell therapy for neurodegenerative disorders like Parkinson's disease (PD). For such therapy, the sources of NPC are genetically unrelated, leading to potential rejection of the transplanted cells by the host immune response. Although numerous studies demonstrate a lack of immunogenicity of mouse ESC and their progenitor derivatives, very few data were reported regarding the potential immune response to human ESC. In preliminary study, we analyzed *in vitro* the allogenic immune response of T lymphocytes and Natural Killer (NK) cells against different sources of NPC. We demonstrated that NK cells induce a strong cytotoxic response to NPC. This response is unrelated to MHC I expression and mainly mediated by NKG2D. To prevent this immune response we tested several immunosuppressive drugs already used empirically in the clinical studies with human fetal NPC. We also demonstrated that cyclosporine and dexamethasone are not only unable to prevent NK alloreactivity but strongly inhibit the terminal differentiation of NPC into mature neurons. We have concluded that immunosuppressive therapy should be carefully considered in the context of allogenic transplantation of human NPC before to envisage their usage in clinical studies.

Immunosuppressive drugs will be necessary to prevent graft rejection. The good regimen should combined the ability to inhibit the T and the NK cells response without interfering with the NPC differentiation into mature neuron.

15:25–15:40

GENERATION OF KIT-EGFP ES AND EG CELLS

Florencia Barrios, Raffaele Geremia, Susanna Dolci
Department of Public Health and Cell Biology, University of Rome Tor Vergata, Rome, Italy

Embryonic and post-natal development transgenic lines carrying the EGFP gene under the control of different regions of the c-kit genomic locus have been previously described (Cairns et al., Blood (2003) 102:3954). We used these transgenic lines to study the expression of c-kit in early embryogenesis, in embryonic stem (ES) cell and embryonic germ (EG) cell generation. In line p13, which carries EGFP driven by 6.9 kb of the c-kit promoter region, EGFP was expressed only in primordial germ cells (PGCs) from 7.5 days post coitum (dpc) on. In line p18 which has, in addition to the p13 construct, 3.5 kb of the first c-kit intron; a faint EGFP positivity was observed at 4–5 cells of the morula stage and maintained at the blastocyst stage in some cells of the inner cell mass (ICM). In line p70, which carries EGFP driven by the p13 construct and 10 kb of the first c-kit intron, embryos showed a faint EGFP positivity in all cells of the morula stage that was maintained in all cells of the ICM of the blastocyst. EGFP expression was studied also during the induction of ES from lines p18 and p70. ICMs from line p18 showed a small group of cells expressing EGFP during the first day of culture. In line p70, all cells of the ICMs showed EGFP positivity. At day 7 of culture, EGFP positive cells with features of ES cells colonies appeared. EGFP was mainly located in the nuclear compartment of the cells, due to the nuclear localization signal contained in the transgenic construct. After establishment of monoclonal EGFP-ES cultures, we found several EGFP negative cells within a single EGFP-ES positive colony. This salt and pepper morphology was maintained in all the colonies. Flow cytometric analysis of these colonies revealed three different cell populations: EGFP strongly positive, EGFP faint and dull types. By western-blot analysis a positive correlation between the levels of the stemness markers

Nanog, Sox-2, and Oct-4 and EGFP was found. In embryoid bodies generated from EGFP positive colonies, EGFP expression was maintained only in the inner part of the aggregates. Derivation of ES and EG cells from all the transgenic lines in the presence of 2i (Mapk and Gskβ inhibitors) resulted in the formation of homogeneus colonies of strongly EGFP positive cells by increasing the expression of Sox2 and Oct4 but not of Nanog. These studies indicate that the c-kit promoter is active very early during embryogenesis, that its activity is maintained during ES and EG derivation, and that it is tightly regulated by Oct4 and Sox2. Furthermore, our observations indicate that transition from unipotency to pluripotency, which occurs when culturing PGCs in 2i, is mediated by a robust increase of the two stemness factors.

15:40–16:00   Disputatio
16:00–16:30   Coffee Break

16:30–16:45

COOPERATION OF BIOLOGICAL AND MECHANICAL SIGNALS IN MURINE CARDIAC PROGENITOR CELL DIFFERENTIATION

Stefania Pagliari, Ana Cristina Vilela-Silva, Giancarlo Forte, Francesca Pagliari, Corrado Mandoli, Stefano Pietronave, Eugenio Magnani, Giorgia Nardone, Giovanni Vozzi, Arti Ahluwalia, Enrico Traversa, Maria Prat, Marilena Minieri, Paolo Di Nardo
Laboratory of Cellular and Molecular Cardiology, University of Rome Tor Vergata, Rome, Italy

Cardiac stem cell niche has been defined as a critical microenvironment in which mechano-physical, biochemical and biological factors concur to preserve resident stem cells in their undifferentiated state. The exhaustive identification of such signals remains among the hot topics in stem cell biology. The generation of an artificial niche in vitro relies, in fact, on the definition of the most appropriate biocompatible, biodegradable scaffold that favours, in combination with specific biochemical factors, stem cell growth and differentiation. The mechano-physical features of biocompatible scaffolds elicit *per se* effects on stem cell determination. We show here that 3D scaffolds can enhance the cardiomyogenic potential of cardiac resident Sca-1$^+$ progenitor cells. In particular, we demonstrate that Sca-1$^+$ stem cell differentiation is achieved within a few days when a complex cardiogenic microenvironment is provided by coupling the biological factors arising from neonatal cardiomyocytes and 3D scaffolds that has cardiac-like stiffness. Challenging the cardiac progenitors only with the appropriate tissue-specific scaffolds merely induced the expression of cardiomyocyte-specific proteins without the assembly of sarcomeres, while the complete differentiation of stem cells in co-culture with neonatal cardiomyocytes in conventional 2D conditions required a longer time. In conclusion, our study provides a further and compelling evidence that cardiac progenitor fate can be tuned by a strict combination of biological and physical factors and encourage in vivo studies to investigate the possibility of using 3D poly lactic acid (PLA) scaffolds to fabricate stem cell-derived cardiac patches.

16:45–17:00

IMPLANTATION OF DENTAL PULP STEM CELLS IN ISOLATED RAT HEART IN THE ABSENCE AND IN THE PRESENCE OF REGIONAL ISCHEMIA

Raffaella Rastaldo, Anna Folino, Andrea E Sprio, Federica Di Scipio, Paolina Salamone, Stefano Geuna, Pasquale Pagliaro, Giovanni N. Berta, Gianni Losano
Department of Clinical and Biological Sciences, University of Turin, Turin, Italy

Dental pulp mesenchymal stem cells (DP-MSC) show excellent differentiation potential in response to specific stimuli. In apparent contrast with such a potential, when implanted they are protected against environmental differentiating stimuli by an early compartmentalization.

Since in co-culture with neonatal cardiomyocytes DP-MSC have been seen to differentiate into cardiomyocytes, aims of the present investigation were to identify the main characterizing markers of DP-MSC and to study their early homing in isolated rat hearts either in normal conditions or after regional ischemia.

Adult Wistar male rats were anesthetized with intra-peritoneal injection of ketamine (90 mg/kg) and Xylazine (10 mg/kg) and killed by decapitation. DP-MSC were then obtained from avulsed teeth and characterized with RT-PCR and immunofluorescence. Characterization revealed that DP-MSC express some precursor markers of cardiomyocytes such as GATA-4, Nkx2.5 and MEF2C. RT-PCR also indicated the transcription of β2-adrenergic receptors.

10^6 cells were marked with carboxyfluorescin and implanted in the ventricular apex of Langendorff isolated syngenic rat hearts perfused with oxygenated Krebs-Henseleit buffer. These hearts were obtained from rats killed as described above.

Two groups of hearts were considered: in control group, DP-MSC were implanted after 20 min of stabilization without ischemia, while in ischemic/reperfused group (I/R group) they were implanted after 20 min of stabilization, 30 min of regional ischemia and 5 min of reperfusion.

Four hours after the implantation, the location of DP-MSC was determined in both groups. In the host tissue DP-MSC were identified by their green color due to carboxyfluorescin. In the I/R group the injured area was evidenced by trypan blue staining.

In the control group DP-MSC remained in the site of implantation as round-shaped clusters, while in the I/R group they migrated towards the injured area. Particularly, in the I/R group some DP-MSC were elongated in parallel with cardiomyocytes and showed the presence of connexin-43 on the membrane.

It may be concluded that in the infarcted heart DP-MSC can migrate close to the infarcted area within about 4 hours and possibly integrate with the surviving cardiomyocytes. Moreover the transcription of β_2-adrenergic receptors suggests that DP-MSC can differentiate not only into myocardial cells but also into coronary smooth muscle fibers.

17:00–17:15

MOLECULAR CHARACTERIZATION OF STEM CELLS IN BREAST CANCER

Gabriella Di Cola, Leopoldo Sarli, Luigi Roncoroni
European Clinic & Research, Emigroup and University of Parma, Parma, Italy

There is experimental evidence of the presence of hallmark stem cell characteristic, such as self renewal, undifferentiated state, and multi-potentiality in a small number of cells in cancer mass. It has earlier been thought that the cancer develops due to the progressive accumulation of random genetic mutations. But these new observations lead to another theory of origin of cancer: that cancer starts from altered adult stem cells. The tumor is considered as an aberrant organogenesis, originated and sustained by these altered stem cells called cancer stem cells or tumor initiating cells. This model had profound theoretical and therapeutic implications. The rogue stem cells can easily evade the action of anti-cancer treatments due to the fact that they can self-renew and are protected from programmed cell death. Their presence in the body can lead to the generation of tumor locally and elsewhere (metastasis). The presence of cancer stem cells and the degree of malignancy in the breast tumor can be determined by characterizing these cells with molecular markers.

In the present study, a panel of molecular markers has been investigated to develop a molecular platform based on a set of validated markers for the detection of stem cells in the breast tumors. A set of known genes, representative of cells that have the ability to self-renew, has been used I in the panel. Characteristic adult stem cell gene expression, with a particular attention to the determinants of asymmetric division, gene markers that are indicative of embryonic origin has been studied. Cells collected from breast cancer biopsies were used in the gene expression study with reverse transcription PCR, and quantitative Real Time PCR, to highlight gene expression of one or more of the following transcription factors: Nanog, Nucleostamin, Oct4, BMI – 1, DPPA4, Stellar, MSI – 1 NUMB, PARD6A, PARD6B, DKK1.

17:15–17:30

IDENTIFICATION OF CIRCULATING KERATINOCYTE PROGENITORS AND THEIR DIFFERENTIATION FOR POTENTIAL APPLICATION IN SKIN TISSUE ENGINEERING
Lissy K Krishnan
Sree Chitra Tirunal Institute for Medical Sciences and Technology, Trivandrum, India

Human peripheral blood mononuclear cell has a mixture of adult stem cells with potential to differentiate in to a wide range of lineages. Bone marrow-derived cells have been reported as transit-amplifying cells at the injured tissue, where they differentiate into keratinocytes. Studies have shown that the bone marrow derived cells could differentiate into a number of different cell types, including epidermis (10). The bone marrow derived stem cells have exhibited capacity to leave bone marrow and circulate in blood (11). A subset of human peripheral blood monocytes behaves as pluripotent stem cells and these cells can be induced to acquire macrophage, epithelial, endothelial, neuronal, and hepatocyte phenotypes (12). The human bone marrow derived mesenchymal cells can differentiate into keratinocyte like cells *in vitro* (13). Sasaki *et al* showed that mesenchymal stem cells are recruited into wounded skin and contribute to wound repair by differentiation into skin cells (14). Medina *et al* reported that circulating bone marrow-derived CD34 positive stem cells might have the capacity to trans differentiate into epithelial-like cells and release matrix metalloproteinase-1-modulating factors (15). They also showed recently that CD14 positive monocytes could to differentiate into keratinocyte like cells (16). Ability of hematopoietic tissue-derived adult stem cells to differentiate into neural progenitor cells offers an alternative to embryonic stem cells as a viable source for cell transplantation therapies to cure neurodegenerative diseases. This approach could lead to the use of autologous progenitors from blood circulation however; due to the limited numbers available, *in vitro* cell expansion may be indispensable.

Previous studies from our laboratory have shown that a fibrin based composite matrix is appropriate for the proliferation and differentiation of endothelial progenitor cells (17). Fibrin which acts as a provisional matrix for the migration and differentiation of cells in wound healing and has been proven to be suitable for various tissue engineering applications (18). In this study we have developed a fibrin based niche and culture condition for the homing, proliferation and differentiation of blood derived circulating stem cells to differentiate into actively dividing keratinocyte cells without the need of any specialized sorting or separating technique. The blood derived stem cells when cultured on fibrin niche expressed p63, a keratinocyte progenitor marker. The ability of these keratinocyte progenitors to differentiate into keratinocytes was analysed by cytokeratin expression. The suitability of these cells to grow on 3D fibrin disc was also analysed. Our results will open a new approach to treat chronic wounds with a tissue engineered skin made of autologous blood derived keratinocyte progenitors grown on autologous plasma derived fibrin matrix.

17:30–17:50   Disputatio
20:00   Visit to the Capitoline Museum Banquet

December 3, 2010

Time: 09:15–13:00
Venue: Round Table, Protomoteca Room, Capitol Hill
Session: Which Strategies to Govern Adult Progenitor Cells Differentiation?
Chair: Yann Barrandon, Ronglih Liao

09:15–09:35

ADULT HUMAN MESENCHYMAL STEM CELLS: CHARACTERIZATION, DIFFERENTIATION, AND APPLICATION FOR HARD AND SOFT TISSUE REGENERATION

Lucy di Silvio
Biomaterials Department, King's College Dental Institute, Guy's Hospital, London, United Kingdom

Demands for clinical status of stem cells warrant validated approaches with guidelines resulting from reproducible experimental data that can form the basis of standardization. Significant efforts have been directed to understanding the factors that influence the lineage commitment of stem cells. Different parameters influence both the rate of growth and behaviour of stem cells and their ability to form specialised tissues with characteristic structure and mechanical properties across the different hierachical scale. This is based on the hypothesis that healthy progenitor cells either recruited or delivered to the injured target site will respond to factors in the mesenchymal stem cell (MSC) environmental niche in the regeneration of new tissue identical to the existing host tissue. *Ex-vivo*, specific attention to media composition, stimulating molecules, in particular cytokines and growth factors, physical and other parameters can influence their metabolic activity and final status.

Objectives

Understand the required cues for directing the differentiation of mesenchymal stem cells (MSCs) towards osteogenesis and chondrogenesis.

Methods

MSCs were isolated from human bone marrow and expanded *in vitro*. Multipotential characteristics were exploited; appropriate environment and chemical signals (TGF-beta or BMP-7) for terminal differentiation and formation of 3-dimensional tissue structures were applied.

Results

A difference in the growth and phenotypic expression marker profiles of MSC's differentiated with TGF-β1 and TGF-β3 was observed. Osteoprogenitor cells expressed osteoblastic characteristics and mineralization in response to environmental and biological cues.

Conclusion

Terminal differentiation of MSCs towards chondrogenic and osteogenic lineage has been demonstrated. For successful implementation of this technology, an integrated contribution is required from MSCs, dynamic culture conditions and 3D scaffolds.

This paper will address the above issues with specific examples of applications.

09:35–09:55

CARDIAC iPS CELLS REPAIR AND REGENERATE INFARCTED MYOCARDIUM

Dinender K. Singla
College of Medicine, Biomolecular Science Center, University of Central Florida, Orlando, USA

Cardiac myocyte differentiation reported thus far is from iPS cells generated from mice and human fibroblasts. However, there is no article on the generation of iPS cells from cardiac ventricular specific cell types. Therefore, whether transduced H9c2 cells, originally isolated from embryonic cardiac ventricular tissue, will be able to generate cardiac iPS cells and have the potential to repair and regenerate infarcted myocardium, remains completely elusive. We transduced H9c2 cells with four stemness factors; Oct3/4, Sox2, Klf4, and c-Myc, and successfully reprogrammed them into iPS cells. These cardiac iPS cells were able to differentiate into beating cardiac myocytes and positively stained for cardiac specific sarcomeric α-actin and myosin heavy chain proteins. Following transplantation in the infarcted myocardium, they differentiated to cardiac myocytes and formed gap junction proteins at 2 weeks post-MI, suggesting that the newly formed cardiac myocytes were integrated into the native myocardium. Furthermore, transplanted iPS cells significantly ($p < 0.05$) inhibited apoptosis and fibrosis and improved cardiac function compared with MI and MI+H9c2 cell groups. Moreover, our iPS cell derived cardiac myocyte differentiation in vitro and in vivo was comparable to embryonic stem cells in the present study. Therefore, we report for the first time that we have cardiac iPS cells which contain the potential to differentiate into cardiac myocytes in the cell culture system and repair and regenerate infarcted myocardium with improved cardiac function.

09:55–10:10

THE PRELIMINARY PORTRAYAL OF A NOVEL CELL-LINE MODEL SYSTEM FOR MOUSE CARDIAC STEM/PROGENITOR (CSC/CPC) CELLS

Ana Freire, Diana S Nascimento, Giancarlo Forte, Isabel Carvalho, Paolo Di Nardo, Perpetua Pinto do O'
Instituto Nacional de Engenharia Biomédica, Universidade do Porto, Porto, Portugal

The view of the adult-heart as a terminally-differentiated organ has been challenged with reports of *de novo* cardiomyocyte generation and the identification of putative cardiac stem/progenitor cells (CPCs). Despite the unknown ontogenic origin of CPCs, commitment to cardiac lineages has been tracked back to a myocardium scarce cell fraction(s) display-ing the stem-cell associated markers Sca-1 and/or c-Kit/MDR1. The rationale for this work is to address whether an immortalized line of Sca-1+ CPCs is a representative *in vitro* model of the native counterparts. A preliminary characterization of the Sca-1+ CPC-line will be presented. Briefly, the CPC-line consistently expressed early cardiac transcription factors and stem-cell associated molecules while no transcripts characteristic of mature car-diomyocytes were found. Markers of hematopoietic and endothelial affiliation were absent as shown by FACS. Upon subcutaneous implant into *Nude* mice cells were detected, up to 14 weeks post-injection, contained within lumps that developed at the injection site. Immuno-histochemical analysis highlighted a vigorous response from the host, likely a result of cell recruitment induced by the grafted-cells. CPCs were not detected in immunocompetent mice on the same experimental setting. The CPC-line response to the native cardiac environment has been evaluated following intramyocardial injection into sham-operated and myocardial-infarcted syngeneic mice. CPCs were identified in the sham hearts at 21 days post-transplant and, despite the profound modifications on the cardiac architecture, were also detected in the infarcted tissue. Examination on how the transplanted cells integrate/interact with the recipient cardiac cells is underway. Validation of the herein cell-line as CPC-representative would entail the first described model for CPCs and thus a tool for dissecting cardiac cell-fate, a source for high throughput molecular analysis and a valuable platform for pharmacological screening.

10:10–10:25

STRATEGIES TO ASSIST CELL DIFFERENTIATION, GROWTH AND DIRECTION FOR TISSUE ENGINEERING

Laura Teodori, Dario Coletti, Maria Cristina Albertini, Marco Rocchi, Massimo Fini and Luigi Campanella
ENEA (Agenzia per le Nuove Tecnologie, l'Energia e lo Sviluppo Economicamente Sostenibile) Roma

Regenerative medicine needs strategies to properly assist stem and precursor cells differentiation, growth and direction arrangement. Our team, at the National Agency for New Technology Energy and the Environment in Italy has previously demonstrated that low intensity static magnetic field (SMF) is able to affect cell growth direction of nerve cells in culture. In a recent paper we demonstrate that SMF, without any invasive manipulation, promotes cell differentiation and hypertrophy, increasing cell fusion efficiency without effecting cell proliferation of myogenic cells. SMF induces myogenic cells to align in parallel bundles, an orientation conserved throughout differentiation. A momentous effect of SMF is the rescue of muscle differentiation in the presence of TNF, a potent muscle differentiation inhibitor, bestowing this feature with important therapeutic implications The SMF-enhanced parallel orientation of myotubes is relevant to tissue engineering of a highly organized tissue such as skeletal muscle. Ideally, the ability to obtain muscle precursor cells (MPC) from a biopsy, growing them for a relatively short period of time and performing autografts of cells with enhanced regenerative capacity is a gold standard.

The recent evidence that intra-arterial delivery of mesoangioblasts corrects the dystrophic phenotype in a mouse model of limb-girdle muscular dystrophy opens new perspectives for the application of stem cell-based therapy. The need to characterize, purify, and amplify large number of muscle precursor cells for cell therapy approaches is becoming more and more pressing. So far, this approach has been characterized by poor efficiency, low functional recovery or immune reaction. The general goal of this study is to develop novel strategies for cell-based therapy and functional recovery of wasting skeletal muscle mainly through the use of SMF: 1) characterize the effects of SMF on muscle differentiation in vitro and in vivo; 2) evaluate whether SMF may affect the behaviour of MPC in transplant studies; 3) characterize the presence of an inflammatory response during the wasting of skeletal muscle and the effects of SFM in the activation of a reparative pathway toward the recovery of the muscle cell function.

10:25–10:40

OSTEOBLASTIC DIFFERENTIATION IN A SUBPOPULATION GEO-GR CD45+ STEM CELL-LIKE BY RAPAMYCIN TREATMENT

Gabriella Marfè, Carla Di Stefano, Valentina Martini, Paola Sinibaldi-Salimei, Marco Ranalli, Alessandra Gambacurta
Department of Experimental Medicine and Biochemical Sciences, University of Rome Tor Vergata, Rome, Italy

Objective

Studies have shown that the phosphoinositide 3-kinase (PI3K) pathway plays important roles in proliferation, survival and maintenance of pluripotency in human embryonic stem cell (hESCs) Inibition of mammalian target of rapamycin (mTOR) signalling by rapamycin suppresses the proliferation of mouse embryonic stem cells (mESCs). Rapamycin's contribution to osteogenic differentiation has been demonstrated in various cell types, but the effect of rapamycin on the osteogenic differentiation of hESCs has not been addressed to date.

In this study, we showed that the treatment with rapamycin (a mTOR inhibitor) induced osteoblastic differentiation in subpopulation stem cell like CD45+, (obtained from getifinib resistant GEO colon cell line GEO-GR). In addition, we report that the mTOR inhibitor rapamycin is capable of differentiating this cells toward an osteoblastic phenotype by blocking p70S6K.

Methods

GEO colon carcinoma cell lines were obtained from the American Type Culture Collection. GEO-GR (Gefitinib resistant), cells were established as previously described (Bianco *et al.*, 2008). – Stem cell like CD45+ subpopulation were selected from GEO-GR by sorting on a BD FACSAria II flow cytometer.

Results

The subpopulation of stem cells like CD45+, obtained from GEO-GR was cultured in osteogenic differentiation media containing rapamycin at the concentration $10 \mu M$. After seven day of culture, 90% of cells presented typical osteoblastic cell morphology, as shown by the expression of osteoblastic marker protein (osteocalcin). Lysates from undifferentiated stem cells like CD45+ (GEO-GR) and inhibitor-treated stem cells like CD45+ (GEO-GR), were analyzed by western blotting using antibodies against p70S6K, phospho-p70S6K (p-p70S6K), and β-actin (as a loading control). Results showed that undifferentiated stem cells like CD45+ expressed active components of the mTOR pathway, such as p-p70S6.

Conclusion

We conclude that inhibition of PI3K-AKT-mTOR signaling by rapamycin contributes to stem cells like CD45+ (GEO-GR) commitment into osteoblastic lineages in vitro and, therefore, present rapamycin as a new osteogenic factor that stimulates the osteoblastic differentiation of this kind of stem cells.

References

1. Bianco R, Rosa R, Damiano V, Daniele G, Gelardi T, Garofalo S, Tarallo V, De Falco S, Melisi D, Benelli R, Albini A, Ryan A, Ciardiello F, Tortora G. (2008). Vascular endothelial growth factor receptor-1 contributes to resistance to anti-epidermal growth factor receptor drugs in human cancer cells. *Clin Cancer Res* 14: 5069–5080.
2. Lee KW, Yook JY, Son MY, Kim MJ, Koo DB, Han YM, Cho YS. (2010). Rapamycin promotes the osteoblastic differentiation of human embryonic stem cells by blocking the mTOR pathway and stimulating the BMP/Smad pathway. *Stem Cells Dev* 19: 557–568.

10:40–11:00   Disputatio
11:00–11:30   Coffee break

11:30–11:45

CHARACTERIZATION OF EPITHELIAL STEM CELLS, BIOMATERIALS AND IN VITRO MICROENVIRONMENT FOR TISSUE ENGINEERING: APPLICATION IN CUTANEOUS ULCER THERAPY

Umberto Altamura, Federico Di Gesualdo, Matteo Lulli, Sergio Capaccioli
Niguarda Hospital, Milan and Department of Pathology, University of Florence, Florence, Italy

11:45–12:00

CONSIDERATIONS ABOUT THE CONTROLLED REPAIR OF DISEASED RENAL PARENCHYMA AFTER IMPLANTATION OF STEM/PROGENITOR CELLS

Will W Minuth, L Denk
Molecular and Cellular Anatomy, University of Regensburg, Regensburg, Germany

The capability of parenchyma regeneration is limited in patients suffering on acute or chronic renal failure. Due to the shortage of kidney transplants and the limitations in dialysis the implantation of stem/progenitor cells for kidney repair is in the focus of actual research. It is problematic that the regeneration is influenced by inflammatory processes. Thus, the process of inflammation has to be turned into an environment promoting implanted stem/progenitor cells to start regeneration. Further supporting influences include the creation of a suitable extracellular surrounding for spatial development, the administration of suitable morphogenic factors released in a time frame by a drug delivery system and the subsequent control of nephron-specific differentiation. The complex task requires standardization on the level of stem/progenitor cells and in the area of biomaterials and growth factors.

To obtain insights in the developmental capacity of stem/progenitor cells, a powerful in vitro model is essential. In the kidney developing tubules are embedded in an interstitium consisting of both extracellular matrix fibers and specific nutritional fluid. To offer a comparable environment an artificial interstitium was created. The technical solution is to culture stem/progenitor cells between layers of polyester fleece (I7, Walraf, Grevenbroich, Germany). The fibers of the fleece simulate extracellular matrix, while the space between the fibers is accessible for the transport of nutrition and respiratory gas.

Fluorescence microscopy demonstrates that numerous tubules are growing in a spatial arrangement. The tubules exhibit a lumen, polarized cells and a basal lamina. So far, the I7 polyester fleece has provided a perfect surrounding for the development of renal stem/progenitor cells. In conclusion, the current experiments make regeneration visible so that new therapeutic options can be investigated.

12:00–12:15

IMPLANTATION OF CARDIAC STEM CELL-LOADED POLY-LACTIC ACID AND FIBRINOIN SCAFFOLDS INTO NUDE MICE TO EVALUATE POTENTIAL FOR CARDIAC MUSCLE TISSUE ENGINEERING

Valentina Di Felice, Angela De Luca, Claudia Serradifalco, Luigi Rizzuto, Antonella Marino, Gammazza, Patrizia Di Marco, Giovanna Cassata, Roberto Puleio, Lucia Verin, Antonella Motta, Annalisa Guercio, Giovanni Zummo
Dipartimento BIONEC, Università di Palermo, Palermo, Italy

Introduction

The rapid translation of preclinical cell-based therapy to restore damaged myocardium has raised questions concerning the best cell type as well as the best delivery route, and the best time of cell injection into the myocardium. Intra-myocardial injection of stem cells is by far the most-used delivery technique in preclinical studies. We have recently demonstrated that c-Kit positive cardiac progenitor cells are able to organize themselves into a tissue-like cell mass in three-dimensional cultures, and with the help of an open-cell poly lactic acid (OPLA) scaffold, many cells can create an organized elementary myocardium.

Hypothesis

We assessed the hypothesis that synthetic scaffolds designed to deliver cardiac progenitor cells in the infarcted region of the heart may induce a better differentiation into cardiomyocytes.

Methods

For the synthesis of poly-DL-lactic acid (PDLLA) scaffolds, the Poly (D,L lactic acid) (RESOMER® 207, MW = 252 kDa) polimer were used (6.7%) in Dicloromethane/Dimetilformamide (DCM/DMF) 70/30 (v/v). The three-dimensional structure was obtained by salt-leaching, using NaCl crystals as porosity agent (NaCl <224 μm and <150 μm). For the synthesis of fibrinoin scaffolds, degummed silk fibres were dried and dissolved into 9.3 m LiBr water solution (20% w/v) at 65°C for 3h. Scaffolds with different porosities, pore size, and properties were made by freeze-drying and salt-leaching. Scaffolds embedded with collagen I and cardiac progenitor cells were implanted in the subcutaneous dorsal region of athymic Nude-Foxn1^{nu} mice.

Results

Cardiac progenitor cells differentiated into cardiomyocytes in vitro into PDLLA scaffolds in M-199 medium supplemented with 20% FBS within 21 days, while a foreign body reaction was observed in vivo. Some fibrinoin scaffolds did not induce a foreign body reaction.

Conclusions

These three-dimensional cultures may be used in the future as a biodegradable patch for the surgical repair of the heart wall or the infarcted myocardium.

12:15–12:30

CHARACTERIZATION AND HEPATIC DIFFERENTIATION OF SKIN-DERIVED PRECURSORS FROM ADULT FORESKIN BY SEQUENTIAL EXPOSURE TO HEPATOGENIC CYTOKINES AND GROWTH FACTORS REFLECTING LIVER DEVELOPMENT

J De Kock, T Vanhaecke, L Ceelen, J Biernaskie, V Rogiers, S Snykers
Department of Toxicology, Dermato-Cosmetology and Pharmacognosy, Vrije Universiteit Brussels, Brussels, Belgium

The rapid translation of preclinical cell-based therapy to restore damaged myocardium has raised questions concerning the best cell type as well as the best delivery route, and the best time of cell injection into the myocardium. Intra-myocardial injection of stem cells is by far the most-used delivery technique in preclinical studies. We have recently demonstrated that c-Kit positive cardiac progenitor cells are able to organize themselves into a tissue-like cell mass in three-dimensional cultures, and with the help of an open-cell poly lactic acid (OPLA) scaffold, many cells can create an organized elementary myocardium.

Hypothesis

We assessed the hypothesis that synthetic scaffolds designed to deliver cardiac progenitor cells in the infarcted region of the heart may induce a better differentiation into cardiomyocytes.

Methods

For the synthesis of poly-DL-lactic acid (PDLLA) scaffolds, the Poly (D,L lactic acid) (RESOMER® 207, MW = 252 kDa) polymer were used (6.7%) in Dicloromethane/Dimetilformamide (DCM/DMF) 70/30 (v/v). The three-dimensional structure was obtained by salt-leaching, using NaCl crystals as porosity agent (NaCl <224 μm and <150 μm). For the synthesis of fibrinoin scaffolds, degummed silk fibres were dried and dissolved into 9.3 m LiBr water solution (20% w/v) at 65°C for 3h. Scaffolds with different porosities, pore size, and properties were made by freeze-drying and salt-leaching. Scaffolds embedded with collagen I and cardiac progenitor cells were implanted in the subcutaneous dorsal region of athymic Nude-Foxn1^{nu} mice.

Results

Cardiac progenitor cells differentiated into cardiomyocytes in vitro into PDLLA scaffolds in M-199 medium supplemented with 20% FBS within 21 days, while a foreign body reaction was observed in vivo. Some fibrinoin scaffolds did not induce a foreign body reaction.

Conclusions

These three-dimensional cultures may be used in the future as a biodegradable patch for the surgical repair of the heart wall or the infarcted myocardium.

12:30–12:40

A NOVEL BIOREACTOR TO MECHANICALLY STRESS RAT MESENCHYMAL STEM CELLS (MSCs) IN CULTURE

M. Govoni, E. Giordano, C. Muscari, G. Pasquinelli, S. Cavalcanti, C.M. Caldarera, C. Guarnieri
Dept. Biochemistry "G. Moruzzi", University of Bologna, Bologna, Italy

Bioreactors, intended as systems able to maintain a controlled chemical culture environment, play a key role in the construction of cell-based products or biological grafts. In bioreactors used to apply to cells a mechanical stretch, often the stimulation operates in an open loop condition, without an accurate control of the force stressing the cells. To overcome such limitation, we have developed a novel bioreactor able to transfer a controlled pulsating stress to the cells, intended for the commitment of competent cells towards the cardiac/muscle phenotype.

Methods

Bone marrow MSCs were isolated from wild type adult male Wistar rats and were seeded onto selected scaffold (3×2 cm hyaluronan-based woven mesh) at the concentration of $10^\wedge 6$ cells per cm^2. Control cells were cultured on scaffold in conventional static condition during 2 weeks, whereas dynamic experimental test was carried out maintained the cells in standard condition during 1 week and transferring them in the bioreactor during the following week. Dynamic cultured conditions were: beating period of 600 ms, mean stress over the cycle of 10 gr and amplitude of stretching of 2.56 mm. At the end of experiment the cells were examined in light microscopy and protein extracts were submitted by SDS-PAGE and Western blot.

Results and Conclusion

After 7 days of "training" in dynamic condition, we observed a significant difference between MSCs cultured in dynamic condition compared with the cells in static control culture. Two main differential features were scored: the large number and the multilayer organization of cells in the dynamic setting. Moreover, biochemical and ultrastructural analysis of the pseudotissue constructs showed typical markers (alpha-sr-1; alpha-SMA) and morphologic features observed in muscle cells.

Therefore, this bioreactor may represent a new basic research tool in the field of tissue engineering and in the study of stem cells differentiation towards specialized phenotypes.

12:40–13:00   Disputatio
13:00–14.20   Lunch

Time: 14:20–16:00
Venue: Round Table, Protomoteca Room, Capitol Hill
Session: Is it Possible to Formulate Efficient Adult Progenitor Cell Protocols for Clinical Applications?
Chair: Maria Jose Goumans, Jun Li

14:20–14:40

CELLULAR THERAPIES AND REGENERATIVE MEDICINE STRATEGIES FOR DIABETES

Camillo Ricordi, Juan Dominguez-Bendala, Armando Mendez, Xiumin Xu, Carlo Tremolada, Luca Inverardi
Diabetes Research Institute and Cell Transplant Center, University of Miami, Miami, USA

The global impact of diabetes and its unsustainable health care costs are constant reminders of the urgent need for novel strategies to cure and prevent this disease condition, rather than improved treatments that do not affect the progression of the epidemic. In this direction, cellular therapies, stem cells and regenerative medicine could offer an definitive solution and an alternative to pharmaceutical treatments. Adult islet cell transplantation has progressed over the last decade with current trials indicating that it is possible to achieve and sustain insulin independence following an allogeneic islet transplant for over 7 years. The most recent data from the Collaborative Islet Transplant Registry (CITR) sponsored by the NIH indicates that islet cell transplants in the context of T-cell depleting induction immunosuppression can achieve graft survival rates comparable to whole organ, pancreas transplantation alone. Now that the proof of principle has been established, the objective of beta cell replacement and regenerative strategies cannot focus on matching clinical results with those of organ transplantation, while using life-long immunosuppression, as this would continue to limit the potential applicability of these procedures only to patients with the most severe form of Type 1 diabetes (i.e., severe hypoglycemic unawareness). Novel strategies involving local immuno-modulation, immune tolerance induction, and conformal/nano-scale immuno-isolation technologies are actively pursued so that transplantation of insulin-producing cells will become applicable to all patients with insulin requiring diabetes. When these strategies will allow for transplantation without immunosuppression, then everyone will want a transplant of insulin-producing cells and because of the severe limitation imposed by human organ donation, it would be impossible to treat all patients that could benefit from this procedure just based on the few multi-organ donors available yearly (e.g., in the USA 1,700 pancreata are transplanted/year and over 20 million patients would require a transplant). It is, therefore, imperative that we aggressively pursue alternative strategies so that an unlimited source of insulin-producing cells will be secured. In this direction, current approaches include animal cells (xenotransplantation), cord blood, amniotic, fetal and embryonic and inducible pluripotent stem cells which expand the potential of transdifferention and tissue reprogramming technologies, opening the way to the use of autologous adult tissues as a potential source for insulin producing cells. Autologous adult stem cell sources have several potential advantages, including reduced or absent teratogenic potential that limits the applicability of embryonic sources. In this direction, recent data from our group and others indicate that adipose derived stem cells could represent an excellent source which can be easily obtained from the patient's own subcutaneous tissue (e.g., following a mini liposuction) procedure. Modern methods for processing adipose tissue derived cells have been described and initial promising results have been recently published in experimental models where it was indeed possible to transform at least a portion of adipose-derived stem cells into insulin-producing cells. While the preliminary data are encouraging, it is too early to raise any hope beyond a level of cautious optimism. Nevertheless, we are confident that cell-based therapy and regenerative medicine strategies will play a critical role in cure-focused strategies for diabetes. While the ultimate source of stem cells is yet to be defined, it is critically important that scientists worldwide continue to explore the potential of different sources of stem cells and related technologies, until the best unlimited source of insulin producing tissue for treating human diabetes will be defined.

14:40–15:00

ADULT STEM CELLS FOR CARDIAC REPAIR AND REGENERATION: PROMISES AND CHALLENGES

Ronglih Liao
Cardiac Muscle Research Laboratory, Brigham and Women's Hospital and Harvard Medical School, Boston, USA

The heart has long been felt to be a terminally differentiated organ with a fixed number of functional cells. As such, any injury resulting in the loss of cardiac muscle cells was believed to be irreversible. Recently, emerging data in both animal models and humans has challenged our prior dogma and demonstrated that the adult heart may be endowed with regenerative capacity. As we know, stem cells have the remarkable ability to renew and differentiate into many specialized cell types in the body when needed. As such, with the current advances in stem cell biology, regenerative medicine has evolved to become an appealing therapeutic strategy for various diseases, including cardiovascular disease. The presentation will focus on adult stem cells, specifically adult resident cardiac stem cells and bone marrow derived stem cells, and their role in repairing and regenerating damage heart tissue. It will aim to provide you with a general overview of the current state of adult stem cell biology and the molecular mechanisms that potentially regulate their adult stem cell fate decision as well as highlight their exciting potential and limitations in cardiovascular regeneration.

15:00–15:20

FEASIBILITY OF ALLOGENEIC BONE MARROW CELLS FOR CELL THERAPY TO REPAIR DAMAGED MYOCARDIUM AFTER MYOCARDIAL INFARCTION

Ren-Ke Li

Department of Cardiovascular Surgery, Toronto General Research Institute, Toronto, Canada

Allogeneic bone marrow mesenchymal stem cells (MSC) are currently undergoing clinical trials to test their potential to repair the heart after a myocardial infarction (MI). Accumulated pre-clinical evidence demonstrates that MSCs can improve cardiac function and may also be immunoprivileged (suitable for allogeneic applications). However, neither the host immune responses nor the fate of implanted allogeneic cells has been investigated. We evaluated the effects of MSC differentiation on the cells' immune characteristics *in vitro* and *in vivo*, and monitored cardiac function for 6 months after post-MI MSC therapy.

Methods and Results

In vitro: The MSCs induced with 5-azacytidine or cytokines acquired myogenic, endothelial, or smooth muscle characteristics. The differentiated cells increased major histocompatibility complex (MHC)-Ia and -II (immunogenic) expression and reduced MHC-Ib (immunosuppressive) expression, and have greater cytotoxicity with allogeneic leukocytes. *In vivo:* The allogeneic or syngeneic MSCs were implanted into infarcted rat heart. At 1 week post implantation, cell survival was similar between the two groups. At 5 weeks after delivery, allo-antibodies against allogeneic MSCs were detected in allogeneic group and implanted MSCs were detected only in the syngeneic group. MSCs (vs. media) significantly improved ventricular function for at least 3 months after implantation. However, functional benefits in allogeneic group were lost within 5 months.

Conclusions

Allogeneic MSC transplantation produced a robust cardiac functional improvement. However, the long-term ability of allogeneic MSCs to preserve function in the infarcted heart is limited by a biphasic immune response, whereby they transition from an immunoprivileged to an immunogenic state following differentiation, which is associated with an alteration in MHC immune antigen profile.

15:20–15:40

GENERATION OF SCAFFOLDLESS HUMAN CARDIAC PATCHES USING ADULT CARDIAC PROGENITOR CELLS AND THERMO-RESPONSIVE TECHNOLOGY

Giancarlo Forte, Stefano Pietronave, Francesca Pagliari, Stefania Pagliari, Eugenio Magnani, Giorgia Nardone, Cristina Giacinti, Antonio Musarò, Enrico Traversa, Teruo Okano, Andrea Zamperone, Marilena Minieri, Maria Prat, Paolo Di Nardo

Laboratorio di Cardiologia Molecolare e Cellulare, Università di Roma "Tor Vergata", Roma, Italy

Stem cells represent a promising tool to treat cardiac pathologies. Nevertheless, the direct injection of stem cells within the myocardium generated poor results, since most of the injected cells were washed away by cardiac contractile activity. On the other hand, using stem cells in combination with polymeric scaffolds, which has been proven effective in hard tissue repair, presents some criticisms due to scaffold degradation rate and byproducts. In this context, thermo-responsive surface technology displays clear advantages since it allows the preparation of scaffoldless, mono- and multilayered bio-constructs overcoming the problem of scaffold removal and by-product release. Moreover, such approach allows the preservation of cell-specific extracellular matrix after cell sheet detachment. Human cardiac Sca-1+ progenitor cells were isolated from atrial auricles after informed consent and used to prepare mono- and multilayered cardiac patches. Cells were grown onto poly-N-isopropylacrylamide (PNIPAAm) thermo-responsive surfaces to prepare scaffoldless stem cell-derived patches. A thorough characterization performed by means of immmunofluorescence, semi-quantitative RT-PCR and microarray techniques demonstrated that cardiac resident Sca-1+ cells can be used to prepare undifferentiated cardiac patches in which cells are functionally connected with each other and preserve their putative phenotype and extracellular matrix. When implanted in vivo in immunosuppressed animals, human cells were found to migrate towards host myocardium and engraft to patches can be fabricated in vitro, thus paving the way to autologous stem cell transplantation into diseased hearts.

15:40–16:00   Disputatio
16:00–16:20   Coffee Break

16:20–16:40

LIMBAL STEM-CELL THERAPY AND LONG-TERM CORNEAL REGENERATION
Graziella Pellegrini
University of Modena-Reggio Emilia, Modena, Italy

Corneal renewal and repair are mediated by stem cells of the limbus, the narrow zone between the cornea and the bulbar conjunctiva. Ocular burns may destroy the limbus, causing limbal stem-cell deficiency. We investigated the long-term clinical results of cell therapy in patients with burn-related corneal destruction associated with limbal stem-cell deficiency, a highly disabling ocular disease.

Methods

We used autologous limbal stem cells cultivated on fibrin to treat 112 patients with corneal damage, most of whom had burn-dependent limbal stem-cell deficiency.

Clinical results were assessed by means of Kaplan–Meier, Kruskal–Wallis, and univariate and multivariate logistic-regression analyses. We also assessed the clinical outcome according to the percentage of holoclone-forming stem cells, detected as cells that stain intensely (p63-bright cells) in the cultures.

Results

Permanent restoration of a transparent, renewing corneal epithelium was attained in 76.6% of eyes. The failures occurred within the first year. Restored eyes remained stable over time, with up to 10 years of follow-up (mean, 2.91 ± 1.99; median, 1.93). In post hoc analyses, success — that is, the generation of normal epithelium on donor stroma — was associated with the percentage of p63-bright holoclone-forming stem cells in culture. Cultures in which p63-bright cells constituted more than 3% of the total number of clonogenic cells were associated with successful transplantation in 78% of patients. In contrast, cultures in which such cells made up 3% or less of the total number of cells were associated with successful transplantation in only 11% of patients. Graft failure was also associated with the type of initial ocular damage and postoperative complications.

Conclusions

Cultures of limbal stem cells represent a source of cells for transplantation in the treatment of destruction of the human cornea due to burns.

16:40–17:00

LIMBAL CELL THERAPY FOR OCULAR SURFACE: A SUCCESSFUL MODEL OF REGENERATIVE MEDICINE
Geeta Vemuganti

Translational medicine is often known as "bench to bedside" — by which the biomedical community attempts to move research discoveries from the laboratory into clinical practice to diagnose and treat patients. One of the emerging fields of translational research is Cell Therapy, most commonly exploiting the potential of stem cells to grow, differentiate and serve the function of the damaged tissue. In ophthalmology, attempts have been made to regenerate ocular surface successfully through cell therapy. The limbus of the eye, a tissue at the junction of the cornea and conjunctiva of the ocular surface is known to harbor the progenitor cells for corneal epithelium hence are extensively used for ocular surface resurfacing in patients with limbal stem cell deficiency. Though clinical use of cultivated limbal epithelium has been in practice more than a decade, the intrinsic and extrinsic factors that govern the growth of these cells is not clearly understood. In an ongoing project approved by the institution IRB, we established a simple, 3T3 feeder-cell free, cost-effective way of culturing the corneal epithelium from limbal tissues within 2 weeks, using human amniotic membrane as a scaffold. Cultivated limbal epithelial cells, at the end of 2 weeks of culture, consisted of a mixed population of stem cell or progenitor cells (ABCG2, p63) progenitor cells and differentiated cells (K3/K12, E-cadherin), with evidence of stratification both in vitro and in-vivo. The interim results of a clinical trial involving 700 patients with severe unilateral and bilateral LSCD revealed 70% success at the end of 3 years, 55–60% at the end of five years. Survival, integration and stratification of the transplanted cells were provided by clinical, histological studies of the corneal buttons obtained from patients who underwent corneal transplantation, status post cultivated limbal epithelial transplantation. Attempts have been made to transplant autologus conjunctiva and to reconstruct the ocular surface but with limited success. Our experience of cultivating the limbal epithelial cell (LEC) on denuded human amniotic membrane using a feeder cell free method, led to identification of mesenchymal like cells of limbus (MLC-L), which showed phenotypic resemblance to bone marrow derived mesenchymal stem cells (MSC-BM). The data shows that these cells are not derived from limbal epithelial cells, rather are derived from limbal stroma within the explanted tissue and bears a striking resemblance to bone marrow derived mesenchymal stem cells (MSC-BM), including the down regulation of human leukocyte antigen DR (HLA DR) expression and the gene expression profile. High expression of certain growth factors (e.g. FGF 1, 2, 7) and their corresponding receptors (e.g. FGFR2) on LECs supports the nurturing roles of the MLC-L.. The lineage specific signatures, evidence of interdependent pathways with limbal epithelial cells, striking resemblance to the signature of bone marrow derived mesenchymal cells support our hypothesis that the limbal stromal cells act like intrinsic feeder cells or the nurture cells, and could possibly be an important component of limbal niche. Thus use of cultivated limbal epithelial cell transplantation for severe ocular surface disease can be considered as a successful model of cell therapy that fulfills the prerequisites for cell therapy, i.e. the desired cells can be grown in sufficient amounts, survive, integrate, network with the host tissues with functional recovery and cause no harm to the recipient. It also led to identification of stromal cells that could possibly be the niche cells of limbal stroma.

17:00–17:20

RESURGENCE OF DORMANT CANCER IS AN IMPERATIVE CONSIDERATION IN STEM CELL THERAPY

Shyam A Patel, Sarah A Bliss, Meneke A Dave, Pranela Rameshwar
Dept of Medicine-Hematology/Oncology, New Jersey Medical School, Newark, USA

Indications for stem cell therapy include, but are not limited to cell replacement/regeneration, halting of further damage to injured tissue, drug or gene delivery, and other method to 'reset' physiological processes. The evidence of embryonic and similar stem cells developing into tumors is evident. However, the unintended consequence of therapeutic source of adult stem cells supporting existing unidentified tumors has not been seriously considered. We have studied the mechanism of dormancy by breast cancer cells. The model can explain a possible mechanism by which stem cells can trigger otherwise dormant cancer cells into highly aggressive tumors. Breast cancer can exist for up to 10 years before clinical detection. During this period, the cancer cells are in dormant phase. Similarly, breast cancer cells can adapt dormancy during cancer remission. Mesenchymal stem cells (MSCs) have evolved as relevant stem cells in the support of breast and other cancers. We have identified breast cancer stem cells as the subset that is protected by MSCs. This occurs partly through direct cellular communication between MSCs and breast cancer stem cells. The two cell types interact by receptor (CXCR4/CXCR7) ligand (CXCL12) and also, through gap junction intercellular communication (GJIC). Consequent to the double interaction is the induction and expansion of regulatory T-cells and exchange of microRNA. In contrast, breast cancer progenitors exhibit weak interaction with MSCs; instead, the cancer progenitors proliferated with concomitant expansion of T-helper 17 that support the growth of the progenitors. The implication for the role of MSCs with respect to stem cell therapy is the high possibility of triggering dormant breast cancer stem cells to metastatic cells. Moving forward, stem cell treatment needs to consider undiagnosed cancer and/or history of cancer in patients. This would require careful treatment design with the oncologists.

17:20–17:35

IMMORTALIZED BONE MARROW-DERIVED MESENCHYMAL STROMAL CELLS PROMOTE AXONAL SURVIVAL IN A MOUSE MODEL OF KRABBE'S DISEASE

Caterina Miranda, Carla Teixeira, Marcia Liz, Vera Sousa, Filipa Franquinho, Giancarlo Forte, Paolo Di Nardo, Perpetua Pinto do O', Monica Mendes Sousa
Nerve Regeneration Group, Institute for Molecular and Cell Biology, Porto, Portugal

In Krabbe's disease, a lysosomal demyelinating disorder, it is essential to devise add-on strategies targeting the peripheral nervous system, as it is not corrected by the existing therapy, i.e. bone-marrow transplantation. We assessed whether intravenous delivery of EGFP+ bone marrow-derived murine mesenchymal stromal cells, immortalized by transfection with telomerase reverse transcriptase (BM-MSCTERT-EGFP), is beneficial in a model of Krabbe's disease, the Twitcher mouse. BM-MSCTERT-EGFP retained the phenotype and multipotency of primary BM-MSC without leading to tumour formation upon transplantation. EGFP+Sca1+ undifferentiated cells grafted the sciatic nerve of transplanted Twitchers at low density. These nerves had a 2.5-fold increase in supporting glia, namely non-myelinating Schwann cell precursors, which likely contributed for the 2.5-fold increased density of unmyelinated axons. To further investigate the neurotrophic effect of BM-MSCTERT-EGFP, the cell line was i.v. delivered to WT mice following sciatic nerve crush. In this model, BM-MSCTERT-EGFP specifically homed to the injured sciatic nerve and increased the number of regenerating axons. In a co-culture system, BM-MSC-TERT-EGFP led to a significant increase in neurite outgrowth, even in the presence of psychosine, the toxic substrate that accumulates in Krabbe's. In vitro, the neuritogenic effect of BM-MSCTERT-EGFP was partially blocked by k252a, an antagonist of the tyrosine kinase family of neurotrophin receptors, and by anti-brainderived neurotrophic factor. In summary, BM-MSCTERT-EGFP i.v. transplantation promotes axonal survival/outgrowth through a paracrine mechanism involving not only the direct secretion of neurotrophins but also the induction of proliferation of Schwann cell precursors. As such, MSC should be considered as an add-on option to bone marrow transplantation in Krabbe's disease and in other disease states that induce axonal loss following demyelination.

17:35–17:45

PRELIMINARY STUDIES ON THE PRODUCTION OF CANINE MESENCHYMAL STEM CELLS FROM ADIPOSE TISSUE AND POSSIBLE APPLICATIONS IN DOGS WITH ORTHOPAEDIC LESIONS

Patrizia Di Marco, Valentina Di Felice, Giuseppa Purpari, Vincenza Cannella, Samanta Partanna, Santina Di Bella, Annalisa Guercio
Istituto Zooprofilattico Sperimentale della Sicilia "A. Mirri", Palermo, Italy

The aim of this study is to evaluate clinical applications in veterinary orthopaedics of canine Adipose tissue Derived Stem Cells (ADSCs) for the treatment of some orthopaedic lesions in the dog. ADSCs are isolated, amplified, characterized and stored. Cells are used in order to study tissue remodelling in both autologous and allogeneic implantation.

Methods

Before implanting the ADSCs, the orthopaedic lesion is clinically evaluate (site, size and severity of the injury). The ADSCs are obtained collecting subcutaneous or visceral fat from the same dog (autologous implantation) or from healthy donor dogs (allogeneic implantation). The identity of the Mesenchymal Stem Cells (MSCs) is verified by their ability to attach to the plastic surface of culture flasks, to form colony-forming units (CFU) and to differentiate in cells derived from mesodermal lineages: chondrocytes, adipocytes and osteocytes. Cells are tested for the expression of specific MSCs markers and the absence of hematopoietic lineage markers. The presence of transcription factors indicative of self-renewal and undifferentiation is also investigated. Moreover, MSCs are tested for possible contaminations (bacteria, fungi, mycoplasma, and viruses) during the steps of production (Quality Controls). Finally, the ability of produced MSCs to induce tumor "*in vitro*" and "*in vivo*" is evaluated. The cells produced are inoculated in dogs with orthopaedic lesions using Platelet Rich Plasma (PRP) or hyaluronic acid as a scaffold.

Results and Conclusion

Regenerative medicine is a new interdisciplinary sector aimed at repairing, replacing, restoring and regenerating damaged tissues and organs through the use of cells that have been manipulated "*ex vivo*". Preliminary results have shown significant clinical improvement of treated dogs. After implantation of MSC, a prolonged follow-up will indicate the real therapeutic capacity of MSCs.

17:45–17:55

DIGGING AND DRAWING CARDIAC PROGENITOR CELL (CPCs) RESPONSE(S) TO HEART INJURY

Diana S Nascimento, M Valente, Ana Freire, S Correia, Isabel Carvalho, Perpetua Pinto do O'
Instituto Nacional de Engenharia Biomédica, Universidade do Porto, Porto, Portugal

Our focus is how stem/progenitor cells (SC) engage in regeneration and repair in adult-tissues. Special emphasis is placed on the mechanisms involved in the regulation of the so-called SC niches. Myocardium-resident putative CPCs display hallmarks of stemness and their antigenic profile, i.e. Sca+/c-Kit+/MDR1+, by matching that of other adult SC, raises the question as to whether CPCs originate in the heart or are continuously replenished from other organs. We address these issues in an integrative manner. An experimental mouse-model of myocardial infarction (MI) was established and the Sca-1+ CPCs have been selected for further analysis. Improvement on the Sca-1+ cell recovery is reported by using the recently released *Gentle-MACS Dissociator*. Isolated Sca-1+ cells display early cardiac-affiliation transcription factors as well as stem-cell associated markers. A majority of cardiac

Sca-1+ cells was found to coexpress CD31 and therefore the population was further separatedinto Sca-1+ CD31+ and Sca-1+ CD31−. Detailed functional and molecular analysis of the two cell-fractions is underway. Furthermore, to portray the CPCs, their differentiating progeny and supporting cells at the natural niche, the optimal reagents/conditions for *in situ* analysis have been identified and, a first drawing of the kinetics of the cardiac-niche's composition following MI is shown. Aiming at the identification of molecules involved in CPCs stress-response signaling pathway(s), and hypothesizing the involvement of Sca-1, expression of the transcript was also evaluated in the Sca-1+ CPCs isolated from non-manipulated, sham-operated and mice subjected to MI. The herein work constitutes a first draft of the molecular blueprint of the CPC response(s) to MI. Identification of the CPC molecular signature and of how cardiac-niche composition is altered in normalcy *vs.* pathology, will contribute knowledge towards *in situ* activation and *ex vivo* amplification of CPCs.

17:55–18:15   Disputatio

Closing Remarks

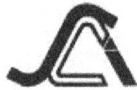

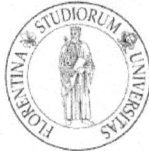

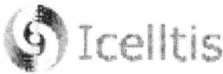

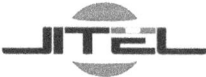

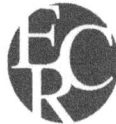

www.ingramcontent.com/pod-product-compliance
Lightning Source LLC
Chambersburg PA
CBHW082113210326
41599CB00033B/6685